VACCINATIONS

VACCINATIONS

Other books in the At Issue series:

VACCINATIONS

Mary E. Williams, *Book Editor*

Daniel Leone, *President*
Bonnie Szumski, *Publisher*
Scott Barbour, *Managing Editor*
Helen Cothran, *Senior Editor*

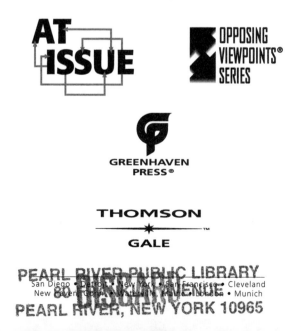

AT **ISSUE**

OPPOSING VIEWPOINTS® SERIES

GREENHAVEN PRESS®

THOMSON
™
GALE

San Diego • Detroit • New York • San Francisco • Cleveland
New Haven, Conn. • Waterville, Maine • London • Munich

THOMSON

━━━━━━✳━━━━━━™

GALE

LIBRARY OF CONGRESS CATALOGING-IN-PUBLICATION DATA

Vaccinations / Mary E. Williams, book editor.
    p. cm. — (At issue)
Includes bibliographical references and index.
ISBN 0-7377-1574-X (pbk. : alk. paper) — ISBN 0-7377-1573-1 (lib. : alk. paper)
    1. Vaccination of children. 2. Vaccination of children—Complications—Risk factors. 3. Immunization of children. 4. Vaccines—Health aspects. I. Williams, Mary E. II. At issue (San Diego, Calif.)
RJ240 .V333 2003
614.4'7'083—dc21   2002032215

Printed in the United States of America

Contents

Introduction

Vaccines are liquid solutions containing dead or weakened forms of infectious microbes that are injected into the body to produce immunity from disease. Vaccinations typically work by inducing the immune system to generate antibodies that attack certain viruses or bacteria. Because the microorganisms contained in vaccines are weak or inactive, their presence can strengthen the body's natural defenses without causing illness. Vaccines also enable the immune system to react quickly and effectively when threatened by disease in the future.

The concept of immunization through inoculation is considered to be one of the most significant advances in scientific history. Western medicine's introduction to the practice most likely occurred in the eighteenth century, when traveling British aristocrat Mary Montagu reported her observations of Turkish children being injected with pus from smallpox victims. Most of these children would contract a mild version of the illness yet later retain a lifelong immunity to it. Similarly, in the United States, Puritan clergyman Cotton Mather learned about vaccination from his African slave Onesimus, who claimed that he had been inoculated with smallpox pus and had never caught the disease. Initially rejected by most Western doctors as a dangerous and barbarous practice, vaccination gained wide support at the turn of the nineteenth century when English physician Edward Jenner created a new smallpox vaccine made from the relatively mild cowpox virus.

During the twentieth century, scientific innovations led to the development of improved vaccines for several infectious diseases. Eventually, as a result of widespread immunizations, previously devastating illnesses such as diphtheria, whooping cough, and tetanus became rare. Smallpox was declared eradicated as a naturally occurring illness in 1980, and polio is expected to be abolished globally during the first decade of the twenty-first century. Most health experts also believe that the eradication of measles is possible.

Despite the general improvement in public health that has resulted from the practice of immunization, the issue of mandatory vaccination has become somewhat controversial in recent years. In the United States, most state laws require children to receive several doses of ten different viral and bacterial vaccines before entering kindergarten. As is the case with all medicines, vaccines can cause side effects in some people, including soreness at the injection site, fever, aches, and fatigue. Severe adverse effects, such as allergic reactions, convulsions, shock, and death are also possible but are reported to be statistically rare. It is these adverse reactions, along with the possibility that some reactions can lead to long-term health problems in certain individuals, that have stirred debate during the past decade.

Vaccination critics argue that the serious side effects associated with vaccines have been underreported and rarely researched. Several analysts have conducted studies that suggest that vaccines are a causal factor in chronic disorders such as asthma, autism, epilepsy, diabetes, learning disabilities, immune system dysfunction, and mental retardation. "Instead of epidemics of measles and polio, we have epidemics of chronic autoimmune and neurological disease," states Barbara Loe Fisher, cofounder of the National Vaccine Information Center in Vienna, Virginia. "In the last twenty years rates of asthma and attention-deficit disorder have doubled, diabetes and learning disabilities have tripled, chronic arthritis now affects nearly one in five Americans and autism has increased by 300 percent or more in many states." Fisher and her supporters claim that children with a family history of immune system disorders or other genetic vulnerabilities are more likely to experience severe vaccine reactions that could result in developmental disabilities or chronic illnesses. Vaccine critics contend that these children should not be forced to submit to a "one size fits all" immunization policy—an approach that ignores individual differences to fulfill legal public health requirements. Fisher and others insist that informed parental consent is preferable to legal mandate as a standard for national vaccination policy.

Most public health experts maintain that immunization critics have exaggerated the potential harms of vaccines and argue that the benefits of vaccination greatly exceed the dangers posed by adverse effects. In examining the risks of disease versus the risks of vaccine, the Centers for Disease Control and Prevention (CDC) reports that one out of every three thousand people who contract measles dies, and one out of every three hundred mumps victims develops encephalitis. However, only one out of every million people given the measles/mumps/rubella (MMR) vaccine develops encephalitis or a severe allergic reaction. In addition, several recent scientific studies have found no conclusive evidence linking vaccines to chronic illnesses and developmental disorders. In 2001, for example, the U.S. Institute of Medicine (IOM) conducted a review of current data and rejected claims of a causal relation between the MMR vaccine and autism. "The fact is that a child is far more likely to be seriously injured by one of these diseases than by any vaccine," the CDC states in a report published on its website. "While *any* serious injury or death caused by vaccines is too many, it is also clear that the benefits of vaccination greatly outweigh the slight risk, and that many, many more injuries and deaths would occur without vaccinations." Allowing individuals to decide if and when their child should be vaccinated, medical experts argue, would lower immunization rates and increase the possibility of disease outbreaks that could become epidemics. The CDC maintains that continuing research "will reduce even further the already low risk of serious vaccine-related injury."

Nevertheless, many observers remain concerned about the side effects of vaccines, partly because the recent immunization safety studies have methodological limitations. For example, the scientific experts who took part in the 2001 IOM study warned that they could not absolutely rule out that the MMR vaccine "may contribute to autistic spectrum disorders" because epidemiological reviews [epidemiology is the study of diseases and their spread] lack the precision to assess rare adverse effects. Furthermore, as Seattle immunologist Gerald T. Nepom admits, "in theory . . . a link between vaccines and autoimmune disease is biologically plausible." So, although no connection between vaccines and chronic illness has been established, neither is there evidence that completely *disproves* such a connection, critics point out.

Reflecting the growing skepticism about vaccine safety is the recent debate about the distribution of the smallpox vaccine—one of the riskiest of the licensed vaccines—in the United States. Routine smallpox vaccinations ended in 1972, when immunologists determined that the health risk of the vaccine had exceeded the risk of contracting the virus. The last case of smallpox in the United States had occurred in 1947, and since the vaccine is associated with a certain number of serious side effects—including disfiguring rashes, encephalitis, neurological damage, and death—experts concluded that the virtual eradication of the disease had made smallpox vaccination an unnecessary hazard. However, after the September 11 terrorist attacks on the World Trade Center and the Pentagon and the subsequent anthrax mailings during the fall of 2001, the American public became increasingly concerned about the possibility of smallpox-wielding bioterrorists striking the United States. Since many Americans have never received the vaccine, and since those who were vaccinated prior to 1972 may no longer be immune, a smallpox terrorist attack could be catastrophic. "Smallpox mortality rates in the unvaccinated top 50 percent," reports *Los Angeles Times* staff writer Edmund Sanders. "On the other hand, if the government resumed smallpox vaccines for the entire U.S. population today, an estimated 300 citizens could die of complications and thousands more would have serious health problems."

In October 2001, the U.S. government contracted with Acambis and Acambis-Baxter Pharmaceuticals to produce enough smallpox vaccine to inoculate every American by the beginning of 2003 or soon thereafter. However, in June 2002, the federal Advisory Committee on Immunization Practices (ACIP) assessed the risk of a smallpox attack as low and recommended against vaccinating the general population. The ACIP instead endorses vaccination for selected emergency medical personnel who can be called upon to respond in case of a bioterrorist attack. If such an event occurs, these personnel would distribute the vaccine only to those who come into direct contact with infected people. This technique, known as "ring vaccination," helped health officials tackle naturally occurring global outbreaks of smallpox in the mid–twentieth century.

Some analysts, however, fear that the ring vaccination strategy would be less effective against a deliberate biological attack, particularly in countries with highly mobile populations. "For example," asks Sanders, "if a terrorist infected with smallpox traveled on New York City subways for a week during rush hour, how would health officials be able to track down all potential contacts?" With such a scenario in mind, some public health officials advocate a gradual resumption of smallpox vaccinations for all Americans—excepting small children, who are more susceptible to health complications.

As the controversy over the smallpox vaccine reveals, balancing the risk of vaccinations against the risk of infectious epidemics can be a troublingly complex issue. For the time being, Health and Human Services secretary Tommy G. Thompson has decided to accept the ACIP recommendation of selective smallpox vaccination for medical personnel, establishing this proposal as official U.S. policy. The authors in *Vaccinations: At Issue* examine the debate over smallpox vaccination as well as several other contemporary arguments concerning the safety and effectiveness of vaccines.

1

Vaccinations Under Scrutiny: An Overview

Gretchen Flanders

Gretchen Flanders, an expert on child immunization policy, works for the National Conference of State Legislatures.

Immunization is one of the most significant advances in medical history. Widespread vaccinations virtually eliminated smallpox and polio by the end of the twentieth century; vaccines have also greatly decreased the incidence of measles, mumps, diphtheria, rubella, and meningitis. Yet concerns about the side effects of vaccines have increased even as vaccination has become more prevalent and more successful at preventing infectious disease. For example, some advocacy groups charge that there may be a connection between immunization and chronic ailments such as autism, multiple sclerosis, and diabetes. They maintain that parents should be given more information about the possible dangers of vaccines and be granted the choice of exempting their children from mandatory immunization programs. Children who receive exemptions from vaccination, however, are more likely to contract infectious diseases.

Arkesea was a healthy, active 15-year-old girl living a normal life in North Minneapolis, until she got hepatitis B. Two weeks later, in July 1998, Arkesea died.

Her family remembers a girl who excelled in math and science and dreamed of becoming a doctor. Neither her doctors nor her parents know how she contracted the disease. She wasn't an IV drug user, she wasn't sexually active, and she didn't receive tainted blood.

Unfortunately, Arkesea was one of the approximately 30,000 children infected with the disease that year. Hepatitis B kills 4,000 to 5,000 people in the United States each year, and approximately 220 people receive liver transplants annually to survive the damage done by the disease. The Centers for Disease Control and Prevention (CDC) estimates that in America today, 1.25 million people are chronically infected. A vaccine to prevent

From "Vaccinations: Public Health's 'Miracle' Under Scrutiny," by Gretchen Flanders, *State Legislatures*, March 2000. Copyright © 2000 by the National Conference of State Legislatures. Reprinted with permission.

hepatitis B is available and was required during the 1998–99 school year for attendance at elementary schools in 27 states, the District of Columbia and Puerto Rico.

Terry, a beautiful, healthy infant from Alabama, received his first in a series of oral polio vaccines when he was nine weeks old. Less than 72 hours later he was in the hospital and on a respirator. Six months later he died. Terry was one of about 10 children each year whose polio is caused by the vaccine designed to protect them. At its height in 1952, the polio epidemic crippled 21,269 Americans and claimed 3,145 lives. To prevent this ever happening again, the vaccine is required for attendance at elementary schools in all 50 states, the District of Columbia and Puerto Rico. But to ward off cases like Terry's, the CDC now recommends the safer, injected form instead of the oral vacine, even though it is less effective.

Vaccines are one of the greatest public health achievements in history.

As policymakers, legislators must ask if states should require that all children receive vaccines in order to protect individuals and communities from infectious epidemics, or should parents be allowed to refuse immunizations to avoid rare, but sometimes serious, reactions?

As guardians of the public health, legislators determine which vaccines should be mandated, when they are to be used and what groups will be affected. It's a complicated issue. As immunizations become more effective, the diseases they prevent fade from memory, leaving only the vaccines themselves and their rare side effects in the public consciousness.

Proponents such as public health officials, the CDC, the American Academy of Pediatrics, the Food and Drug Administration and child health advocates point out that serious medical problems caused by vaccines occur very rarely—much more rarely than the serious complications and deaths that can be prevented by vaccines. Numerous scientific studies have failed to draw any correlation between vaccines and autism, Sudden Infant Death Syndrome (SIDS), multiple sclerosis or a number of other diseases.

However, the public sometimes has a hard time believing the experts, as we've seen with the Gulf War syndrome and silicone breast implants—cases where experts tried and failed to establish cause and effect. The public believes the experts just haven't tried hard enough, said John Donvan of *Nightline* in an October 1999 program.

Yet, in our society, pharmaceuticals are tested so stringently that we have devoted an entire federal bureau to the task. In fact, immunizations are subject to a higher standard of safety than other medical interventions because they are given to healthy children. But is this enough?

Public health's role

Vaccines are one of the greatest public health achievements in history. Smallpox has been eradicated worldwide through the use of vaccines. Polio, except for the few cases caused by the vaccine, has been virtually eliminated in the Western Hemisphere and may be eradicated in the rest of the world in the year 2000. Vaccines against measles, diphtheria, mumps, rubella and Hib (one kind of infant meningitis) have decreased the number of cases by more than 99 percent. In 1998, this country had only one reported case of diphtheria and no cases of wild polio.

Former Health and Human Services Secretary Donna Shalala says immunizations are one of the "most cost effective of all preventive public health practices." Wisconsin learned about this the hard way when a 1989 measles epidemic with more than 600 cases claimed the lives of three children and cost the Medicaid program $1.5 million in hospitalizations.

But as they become more effective and the diseases they prevent fade from our memories, the concerns about side effects gain attention. Most parents today don't remember being quarantined with measles or whooping cough; most don't remember the terror of the iron lung.

"Although I don't remember the experience well, I know I was quarantined as a child, and I wasn't allowed to leave the house for a long time," says Senator Grant Ipsen, chair of the Health and Welfare Committee in Idaho. "For a young child, that's a hard thing to accept. I think that some of the young parents today don't know what it was like to see these diseases firsthand. They don't always get a clear picture of what immunizations are protecting them from."

Community immunity?

Vaccination of an individual doesn't just protect that one person, it also guards other members of the community. "Herd immunity allows us to eliminate vaccine-preventable disease without needing 100 percent of the population to be immune," says Dr. Walter Orenstein, director of the CDC's National Immunization Program.

Senator Ipsen knows this benefit well; his grandchildren have immune systems that don't function properly so their vaccinations were delayed, then administered under the close supervision of their doctor. "We had to rely on others to get their vaccinations so that our grandchildren could be protected indirectly until it was safe for them to be immunized," Ipsen says.

"There may be some appeal to the idea that immunizations should be an individual decision, but, because vaccines protect both the individual and the community, decisions about opting out of immunizations have both personal and community implications," says Dr. Bruce Gellin, executive director of the National Immunization Information Network. He compared it to a four-way stop sign. "A person who decides to ignore the stop sign knows he has less risk of an accident if others obey it. However, if two drivers make a similar decision, assuming that the other will stop, the outcome becomes much more risky for everyone in the intersection."

Vaccine safety

Some groups that believe vaccines have caused serious illnesses are not "antivaccine," but they do strongly advocate more exemptions from mandates, more research into the connection between vaccines and side effects, and informed consent from parents.

"What American citizens from all walks of life are telling us is that they don't want Big Brother breathing down their necks and telling them what health care choices to make," says Barbara Loe Fisher, president and cofounder of the National Vaccine Information Center. Dr. Jane Orient of the American Association of Physicians and Surgeons, a conservative medical group, says, ". . . we are concerned that immunization mandates subject patients to medical treatment without their fully informed consent." The risks are not completely known in the absence of long-term safety studies, she contends.

Groups such as these argue that vaccines are not tested enough before mandating coverage and that more research is needed to investigate the connections between immunizations and diseases such as multiple sclerosis and diabetes.

How are vaccines monitored?

Vaccines are monitored through the Vaccine Adverse Event Reporting System to look for rare events that may not show up in clinical trials. The CDC has also created the Vaccine Safety Datalink study that links computerized vaccination records with medical visit records on 6 million members of four health maintenance organizations. This enables the CDC to continuously examine possible associations between vaccines and serious side effects.

The task of monitoring vaccine safety is not an easy one. Because so many developmental and psychological problems are diagnosed at around the same time that kids are getting their vaccines, sometimes the problems are blamed on the vaccine even when it might not be the cause. The scientific way to determine if a vaccine is causing another disease is to compare the disease incidence in children who were vaccinated to those who were not. However, these studies are long, expensive and difficult to design. The data collected through the Vaccine Safety Datalink should help.

As [vaccines] become more effective and the diseases they prevent fade from our memories, the concerns about side effects gain attention.

An example of this continued monitoring was recently seen with the new rotavirus vaccine, developed to prevent one of the most common causes of severe diarrhea in children. After testing and review, the Advisory Committee on Immunization Practice recommended in March 1999 the rotavirus vaccine for infants. In July 1999, the CDC recommended that health care providers stop using the vaccine based on reports that a rare type of bowel obstruction had occurred in 15 recently vaccinated children. Upon subsequent review, the committee withdrew its recommendation for use of the vaccine.

Dr. Bruce Gellin points out that ". . . all along the continuum of vaccine development, we learn about its performance and side effects. Should we withhold a vaccine because we can't confidently say that we know every detail about it? It seems that this is a prescription to do nothing."

Groups that question vaccine safety contend that while vaccines are stringently tested by the FDA, they are not always tested on infants and their effects are not followed for long enough periods of time. They also argue that scientists who are looking for vaccine side effects or who have been known to question their safety are not given funding by the government to conduct research on these issues.

Federal help and oversight

In 1986, Congress passed the National Childhood Vaccine Injury Act in response to concerns about the safety of a particular type of whooping cough vaccine. Negative publicity about the shot occurred in this country and also spread in Japan and the United Kingdom, which led to a serious decline in vaccine coverage. In Japan, where the pertussis vaccination rate fell from 80 percent to 20 percent in 1979, the resulting epidemic caused more than 13,000 cases and 41 deaths. The United Kingdom suffered several whooping cough epidemics, one of which caused more than 100,000 cases and 36 deaths. In this country, pertussis vaccine rate remained high, but numerous lawsuits were filed against manufacturers, which resulted in higher prices for vaccines. Several companies decided to stop production, causing temporary shortages.

The congressional program provides for independent review of the available scientific evidence on adverse effects to vaccinations, mandates the reporting of vaccine-associated problems to the Department of Health and Human Services, provides financial compensation to families affected by side effects and creates the Vaccine Adverse Event Reporting System to monitor vaccine side effects.

State laws and exemptions

Recommendations from the Advisory Committee on Immunization Practice, a federally chartered group, and the Committee on Infectious Diseases of the American Academy of Pediatrics give states the option of passing a law or adding a regulation requiring that a vaccine be administered as recommended for children entering school or day care. No federal laws exist requiring immunization for school or day care entry, although some federal programs tie immunizations to services such as day care subsidies.

State laws requiring immunization have been around since the early 1800s when Massachusetts enacted a smallpox vaccination requirement. Widespread school and day care vaccination laws came about in the 1960s and '70s during the effort to eradicate measles. Specific vaccines and requirements differ from state to state.

All states allow vaccine exemptions for medical reasons. Religious exemptions exist in 48 states, the District of Columbia and Puerto Rico, but not in Mississippi or West Virginia. These laws vary. In Texas, the family must belong to a recognized religious group that opposes all immunizations and must present a letter from a religious leader. California, on the other hand, requires only that a parent sign an affidavit declaring a personal belief against immunization.

Fourteen states allow philosophical or personal exemptions. Overall, less than 1 percent of the population claims exemptions, but this small group can have a dramatic impact on a community. The issue of allowing exemptions is highly controversial.

The *Journal of the American Medical Association* reports that exempted children, who tend to cluster within communities, were 35 times more likely to contract measles than vaccinated children. Several vaccine-preventable disease outbreaks have originated in groups with high numbers of exemptions. In a 1996 measles outbreak in Utah, 45 percent of cases were among families who had claimed exemptions. However, concerned groups believe that parents should be allowed to decide if their children should be vaccinated.

All sides of this debate have the same concerns at heart. They all want children to be healthy and protected. It's just the ways to achieve this goal that are contentious. The fact that vaccines prevent a huge number of illnesses, but have some side effects, makes for a difficult policy question, but not one that hasn't been solved in other areas.

"All states require that children use seat belts or car seats to prevent injuries even though there are certainly instances when wearing a seat belt actually causes more serious injuries or even death. In making decisions about public health issues such as seat belt laws or immunizations, we as policymakers must constantly weigh the public benefits against individual freedoms combined with the newest research to ensure that the policies are providing the largest benefit to the largest group. Immunizations for children clearly fall into this same category," says Representative Marcy Morrison, chair of Colorado's Health, Environment, Welfare and Institutions committee. "Above all, we must make decisions that protect the public health."

2

Vaccines Are Safe and Effective

Michelle Meadows

Michelle Meadows is a staff writer for the FDA Consumer.

Immunization remains humanity's best defense against life-threatening infectious diseases such as whooping cough, influenza, and pneumonia. Moreover, several governmental agencies, including the Food and Drug Administration (FDA), the Centers for Disease Control and Prevention (CDC), and the National Institutes of Health (NIH), consistently monitor vaccine safety and effectiveness and implement new discoveries that create improved vaccines. As is the case with all medicines, vaccines do carry a small risk of serious side effects, including allergic reactions, illnesses, and disabilities; however, the benefits of vaccination far outweigh these risks. Consumers should become well informed about the advantages and drawbacks of vaccines and reject the opinions of alarmists who report inaccurate data and overstate the dangers of immunization.

Smallpox and polio have been wiped out in the United States. Cases of measles, mumps, tetanus, whooping cough (pertussis) and other life-threatening illnesses have been reduced by more than 95 percent. Immunization against influenza and pneumonia prevent tens of thousands of deaths annually among elderly persons and those who are chronically ill. As a result, millions of lives have been saved. But don't let the success of vaccines fool you into thinking we no longer need them. Most vaccine-preventable diseases aren't gone.

Steve Berman, M.D., president of the American Academy of Pediatrics and a pediatrician in Denver, says he and his colleagues were devastated to recently see an infant die of whooping cough. "This was a case where the family thought the risks of vaccination outweighed the benefits," Dr. Berman says. The baby was exposed to the disease by two older brothers who hadn't been vaccinated.

Vaccines contain a weakened (attenuated) or killed (inactivated) form

From "Understanding Vaccine Safety," by Michelle Meadows, *FDA Consumer*, July/August 2001.

of disease-causing bacteria or viruses, or components of these microorganisms, that trigger a response by our body's immune system. For example, vaccines stimulate our bodies to make antibodies—proteins that specifically recognize and target the bacteria and viruses against which the vaccines are designed, and that help eliminate them from the body when we encounter them.

Without vaccine protection, we can easily contract and transmit infectious diseases. It may only take one person, whether it's a family member, a neighbor, or a visitor from another country, to start the spread of a disease. And even immunized individuals can be at risk because no vaccine is ever 100 percent effective for everyone.

Most parents believe in the benefits of vaccination, as evidenced by record high childhood vaccination rates, and more and more adults are getting vaccinated against influenza, pneumococcal disease, and tetanus. But some people who need vaccines don't get them for a variety of reasons, including fear of side effects. Lately, a surge of negative publicity focusing on the risks of vaccines—some of which are unproven or inaccurate—has some wondering whether they do more harm than good. But vaccine experts and the overwhelming majority of health-care providers caution consumers against skipping important vaccinations because of an evening news report or a posting on the Internet.

Don't let the success of vaccines fool you into thinking we no longer need them. Most vaccine-preventable diseases aren't gone.

Sometimes such reports contain unsubstantiated or inaccurate information and don't reflect a balanced view of the risks and benefits of a particular vaccine.

The Food and Drug Administration (FDA) recommends that consumers arm themselves with the facts about the benefits and risks of vaccines, along with the potential consequences of not vaccinating against certain diseases. According to a Washington state–based organization called Parents of Kids with Infectious Diseases (PKIDS), some parents are shocked to learn that children can die of chickenpox and other vaccine-preventable diseases they hadn't considered a threat.

The FDA's Center for Biologics Evaluation and Research (CBER) regulates vaccines in the United States, and works with several other agencies, including the Centers for Disease Control and Prevention (CDC) and the National Institutes of Health (NIH), to study and monitor vaccine safety and effectiveness. New vaccines are licensed only after the FDA thoroughly reviews the results of extensive laboratory studies and clinical trials performed by scientists, physicians, and manufacturers.

For vaccines intended for wide use in healthy populations such as children, clinical testing with careful safety monitoring typically involves thousands of patients before a vaccine is ever licensed. And after a vaccine hits the market, the safety monitoring continues, as does FDA oversight to assure the highest levels of quality control in the vaccine production process.

"We are always monitoring for evidence that might suggest possible problems with vaccines," says Karen Midthun, M.D., director of CBER's office of vaccine research and review. CBER scientists also conduct research to better ensure vaccine safety and to better understand vaccine-related side effects.

A commitment to safety

On the surface, it may seem that approaching vaccine safety as a continuous process—always looking into problems and potential problems—implies that vaccines are unsafe. "But it's actually a reflection of our ongoing commitment to safety, and to assuring the prevention of potentially lethal infectious diseases," says Jesse Goodman, M.D., M.P.H., deputy director for medicine at CBER. "It's also the nature of science to seek and implement improvements which make for safer and more effective medical products."

Since 1996, for example, CBER has licensed several acellular pertussis vaccines. Acellular pertussis vaccines use only parts of the disease-causing bacteria and are associated with fewer side effects than the whole cell pertussis vaccines that had been in use. In 1997, the CDC's Advisory Committee on Immunization Practices (ACIP) recommended a switch from using the whole cell pertussis component of the diphtheria, tetanus, pertussis (DTP) vaccine to using acellular pertussis vaccines for all five doses in the childhood schedule.

The National Institute of Allergy and Infectious Diseases (NIAID) sponsored clinical trials for some of the experimental acellular vaccines. "We set out to develop an improved vaccine that would be as effective as the standard whole cell vaccine but cause less extended crying, fevers, and other side effects," says Carole Heilman, Ph.D., director of NIAID's division of microbiology and infectious diseases. CBER scientists also played a critical role by developing methods to evaluate the acellular vaccines, which helped them get to clinical trials faster.

There have been other recent policy changes to improve vaccine safety, including ACIP's 1999 recommendation to change from the use of oral polio vaccine (OPV) to the inactivated polio virus (IPV). OPV had been highly effective in controlling naturally occurring polio outbreaks, preventing thousands of cases of paralysis a year. But as a live virus, it mutated in extremely rare cases to cause polio itself. Continued use of OPV resulted in about 10 cases of paralytic polio each year among millions vaccinated and their contacts, according to William Egan, Ph.D., deputy director of CBER's office of vaccine research and review. Switching to the use of IPV eliminated this risk and was appropriate once epidemic polio was controlled.

"There are times when we also take action even when there is just the theoretical potential for harm," Goodman says. Thimerosal, a mercury-containing compound, had been the most widely used preservative in vaccines. Its use in minute amounts helped to prevent bacteria from contaminating multi-dose vials of vaccines and other medicines, protecting against potentially serious infections. But thimerosal has been nearly eliminated from vaccines because of legitimate and growing scientific concerns about the possible effects of mercury on the nervous system, Goodman says.

"In addition, as the numbers of vaccines used in children has increased, small infants who received every recommended vaccine could be exposed to cumulative doses of mercury that exceeded some, but not all, federal guidelines," Goodman explains.

Even though there are no convincing data that show harm because of thimerosal in vaccines, the U.S. Public Health Service recommended moving rapidly to vaccines that are thimerosal-free. The FDA encouraged manufacturers to comply and set the highest priority for its reviews of such products, Goodman says. As a result, all recommended pediatric vaccines available are now thimerosal free or have greatly reduced thimerosal contents. In March 2001, the FDA approved a newly formulated version of Tripedia, a diphtheria and tetanus toxoids and acellular pertussis (DTaP) vaccine with only a trace amount of thimerosal.

A thorough process

The most common components of vaccines are weakened microbes (disease-causing microorganisms), killed microbes, and inactivated toxins. In addition, subunit vaccines, which only use a part of the bacterium or virus, are increasingly being used.

Manufacturers conduct stringent tests to make sure that cell lines used for producing viral vaccines do not contain adventitious agents (unwanted viruses) such as simian virus 40 (SV40), which was found in some early polio vaccines. These vaccines had been manufactured in kidney cells from simians (monkeys) that harbored SV40. Following its discovery, SV40 was removed from vaccines, and vaccines have been free of the virus since the early 1960s. CBER scientists are developing potentially better methods to detect such infectious agents.

New vaccines are licensed only after the FDA thoroughly reviews the results of extensive laboratory studies and clinical trials.

Developing vaccines is a thorough and rigorous process, Egan says. Vaccines are tested for safety on animals first, and then in humans during several phases of clinical trials. The most important clinical trial for the recently licensed vaccine Prevnar involved nearly 40,000 people, equally divided between those who received the vaccine and those who did not. Prevnar was approved to prevent invasive pneumococcal diseases such as meningitis.

A group of FDA scientists reviews data and the proposed labeling of the vaccine, which includes directions for use and information about potential side effects. The committee also reviews manufacturing protocols, conducts its own tests, and inspects the manufacturing facility. The FDA's Vaccines and Related Biological Products Advisory Committee, which includes scientific experts and consumer representatives, can be consulted at any time to review data and recommend action to the agency.

After a vaccine is licensed, the FDA generally requires that manufacturers use validated methods to test samples from each vaccine lot for safety, potency, and purity prior to its release for public use. The FDA also tests selected lots and products to help assure the accuracy of tests conducted by the manufacturers.

Common concerns

"Most vaccines cause some side effects, but they are usually minor and short-lived like low-grade fever and soreness at the injection site," Midthun says. Serious vaccine reactions—causing disability, hospitalization, or death—are extremely rare but they can happen.

Like any medicine, vaccines carry a small risk of serious harm such as severe allergic reaction. But experts point out that the risk of being harmed by a vaccine is much lower than the risk that comes with infectious diseases.

For example, in 1976, the swine influenza (flu) vaccine was associated with a severe paralytic illness called Guillain-Barré Syndrome (GBS). According to the CDC's vaccine information sheet on the influenza vaccine, "if there *is* risk of GBS from current influenza vaccines, it is estimated at 1 or 2 cases per million persons vaccinated, much less than the risk of severe influenza, which can be prevented by vaccination." Each year, flu causes tens of thousands of deaths, mostly among older people. Most people who get the influenza vaccine have no serious problem from it.

And though some people worry about it, you can't get the flu from the flu vaccine, Midthun says. "Just as there are no vaccines that are 100 percent safe, there are also none that are 100 percent effective," she says. "So you may get the flu soon after you received the vaccine, before it could be expected to protect you. It does not mean the shot gave you the flu," she says.

Some live virus vaccines, such as the chickenpox vaccine, can cause mild versions of the disease they protect against, says Goodman. "But this is usually only a serious problem if the patient has a severely compromised immune system." And vaccines are generally not advised for such people. It's important to talk with your doctor about the benefits and risks of vaccines, and any concerns you may have, specifically as it relates to you and your family. If you or your child has previously had a significant reaction to a vaccine, that may affect the risk/benefit ratio for the individual and whether that vaccine should be recommended again.

How reactions are evaluated

Before a vaccine is put into standard medical practice, it must be studied in clinical trials of thousands of people, which allows for evaluation of relatively common side effects. For example, a common side effect might occur in one or more of several hundred vaccine recipients. But rare events (fewer than one case in several thousand recipients) aren't usually evident in clinical trials. "Unless you've studied something in a million or more people, you might never see the very rare event or be able to know whether it occurred due to vaccination or simply by chance," Goodman says.

Through the Vaccine Adverse Event Reporting System (VAERS), jointly operated by the FDA and the CDC to monitor the safety of licensed vaccines, experts look for patterns and any unusual trends that may raise questions about a vaccine's safety once it is used more widely in the population. The FDA continuously reviews and evaluates individual reports, in addition to monitoring overall reporting patterns. The FDA also monitors reporting trends for individual vaccine lots. Most reports come from health-care providers, but anyone can report an unexpected event after vaccination to VAERS.

VAERS receives 800 to 1,000 reports each month. Because it often can't be determined whether an adverse event occurring after vaccination was actually caused by the vaccination, health-care providers and consumers are encouraged to report any event that might be attributable to a vaccine.

"You don't have to be sure," says Susan Ellenberg, Ph.D., director of CBER's office of biostatistics and epidemiology. "Reporting possible reactions will help identify adverse events that might be truly associated with vaccinations and need further study." But this approach to reporting means that one can't assume that all VAERS reports describe true vaccination reactions.

VAERS is a passive, voluntary reporting system, which means not all adverse events get reported. It also means that many reports are incomplete or even contain inaccurate information because the forms are not filled out by trained personnel. Another problem with interpreting VAERS data is the lack of information on the total number of individuals who received a particular vaccine, making it impossible to estimate the incidence of reported adverse events. It's also often the case that multiple vaccines are given at the same time, further complicating the interpretation of what might have caused the event, Ellenberg says.

Despite these problems, VAERS does contribute in important ways to understanding vaccine safety. VAERS data may suggest the need for more research on certain vaccines. "In this sense, VAERS is a signal generator," Egan says. Recently, VAERS data were instrumental in evaluating RotaShield, a vaccine licensed to protect against rotavirus infection. Rotavirus is the most common cause of gastroenteritis in children younger than five and can result in severe diarrhea, dehydration, and death. This virus is an especially serious problem in developing nations, where it kills hundreds of thousands of children every year.

The risk of being harmed by a vaccine is much lower than the risk that comes with infectious diseases.

Following the vaccine's licensure, VAERS started to receive reports of bowel obstruction in a number of infants who had received RotaShield. Careful review of these reports revealed that the bowel obstruction occurred most often in the first two weeks after RotaShield was administered. As a result, the CDC recommended postponing any further distribution or administration of RotaShield until more data could be collected and evaluated.

The FDA discussed the concerns with the manufacturer, which decided to voluntarily withdraw the product from use. In November 1999, ACIP withdrew its previous recommendation for universal use of the vaccine. At this time, the FDA, NIH, and CDC are still studying the bowel obstruction and RotaShield-associated cases, Egan says. "We continue to look into mechanisms for any serious adverse events. We want to understand why they happen so that we can prevent them from occurring in the future."

Vaccination is the reason we don't see the suffering, disability, and death from whooping cough, measles, polio and other infectious diseases like we used to.

The CDC's Vaccine Safety DataLink, which links computerized histories of vaccination to hospitalization records and other medical information for members of eight large managed care organizations, supplements the information in VAERS and permits more rigorous evaluation of possible safety concerns. For example, the system allows researchers to compare how often an adverse event occurs in people recently vaccinated with those not recently vaccinated, to evaluate the likelihood that the vaccine caused the adverse event.

Alleged associations

Some have looked to vaccines to explain a host of serious conditions that we don't fully understand, including sudden infant death syndrome (SIDS), multiple sclerosis, diabetes, and autism. There have been a number of epidemiological studies of these possible associations, and experts say there is no good scientific evidence at this time showing that vaccines cause these diseases or conditions.

"Physicians give vaccines to children at multiple time points during their development and a lot can happen during that time," says Midthun. She stresses that both the FDA and the CDC take concerns of parents seriously. After careful review of all available information, neither agency has found that existing data support any link between the measles, mumps, and rubella (MMR) vaccines and autism, a hypothesis that has received considerable publicity over the past few years.

The CDC and the NIH recently contracted with the Institute of Medicine, part of the National Academy of Sciences, to establish the Immunization Safety Review Committee. The independent committee is charged with evaluating nine vaccine safety topics over a three-year span. The possible association of the MMR vaccine and autism was the first topic.

On April 23, 2001, the Immunization Safety Review Committee reported its finding that the current evidence does not favor the hypothesis that there is a link between MMR and autism, and that no changes should be made in the current policy of administering the MMR vaccine. The committee could not rule out the possibility that the MMR vaccine might be linked to autism in some subpopulation, and recommended that targeted research in this area be conducted. To date, there is no indication as to whether there is any such subpopulation, or what the genetic makeup or other characteristics of such a subpopulation would be, Egan says.

"It's important that policy decisions about vaccine safety be based on science," says Martin G. Myers, M.D., director of the U.S. Department and

Health and Human Service's National Vaccine Program Office. As vaccine safety research continues, Myers says, we can't afford to lose sight of what life was like before immunization. Vaccination is the reason we don't see the suffering, disability, and death from whooping cough, measles, polio and other infectious diseases like we used to.

"Vaccines are very safe," Myers adds, "but nothing is without risk." Not vaccinating against certain diseases means choosing another type of risk, he says. Myers recalls treating an infant with seizures from tetanus so strong they shook the baby's whole body. These types of seizures and many deaths are preventable by vaccination. And Myers still has an audiotape from the early eighties of a child hacking and gasping for air because of whooping cough. "The child's mother asked me to play it for parents who might be undecided about getting vaccinated." He's also played the tape for medical students and residents. "It doesn't take long before somebody in the room asks me to please turn it off."

3

Vaccines Are Unsafe and Ineffective

Alan Phillips

At the time of this writing, Alan Phillips was a third year law student attending the University of North Carolina at Chapel Hill, and a co-founder and codirector of Citizens for Healthcare Freedom (CHF), a nonprofit organization dedicated to raising vaccine awareness and advocating informed choice.

Vaccines are neither safe nor effective. Solid research has connected vaccines with adverse effects, including allergic reactions, disabilities, chronic health problems, and death. Moreover, vaccination is not a reliable method of preventing infectious disease— statistics reveal that epidemics have occurred after the introduction of compulsory immunization programs and in populations that have been completely vaccinated. Childhood diseases rarely have serious consequences in the modern world, and exposure to illnesses like measles and mumps may even play a role in enhancing the body's long-term natural defenses. Instead of submitting to mandatory immunization programs, consumers and parents need to educate themselves about the negative effects of vaccines.

When my son was set to begin his routine vaccination series at age 2 months, I didn't know there were any risks associated with immunizations. But the clinic's flyer contained a contradiction: my child's chances of a serious adverse reaction to the diphtheria/pertussis/tetanus (DPT) vaccine were one in 1750, while his chances of dying from pertussis were one in several million. When I pointed this out to the physician, he angrily disagreed, and stormed out of the room mumbling, *"I guess I should read that [flyer] sometime . . ."* Soon thereafter I learned of a child who had been permanently disabled by a vaccine, so I decided to investigate for myself. My findings have so alarmed me that I feel compelled to share them; hence, this report.

Health authorities credit vaccines for disease declines, and assure us of their safety and effectiveness. Yet these assumptions are directly contradicted by government statistics, published medical studies, Food and Drug Administration (FDA) and Centers for Disease Control (CDC) reports, and the opinions of credible research scientists from around the world. In fact, infectious diseases declined steadily for decades prior to mass immunizations, doctors in the U.S. report thousands of serious vaccine reactions each year including hundreds of deaths and permanent disabilities, fully vaccinated populations have experienced epidemics, and researchers attribute dozens of chronic immunological and neurological diseases that have risen dramatically in recent decades to mass immunization campaigns.

Doctors in the U.S. report thousands of serious vaccine reactions each year including hundreds of deaths and permanent disabilities.

Decades of studies published in the world's leading medical journals have documented vaccine failure and serious adverse vaccine events, including death. Dozens of books written by doctors, researchers, and independent investigators reveal serious flaws in immunization theory and practice. Yet, incredibly, most pediatricians and parents are unaware of these findings. This has begun to change in recent years, however, as a growing number of parents and healthcare providers around the world are becoming aware of the problems and questioning mass mandatory immunization. *There is a growing international movement away from mass mandatory immunization.* This report introduces some of the information that provides the basis for the movement.

My point is not to tell anyone whether or not to vaccinate, but rather, with the utmost urgency, to point out some very good reasons why everyone should examine the facts before deciding whether or not to submit to the procedure. As a new parent, I was shocked to discover the absence of a legal mandate or professional ethic requiring pediatricians to be fully informed of the risks of vaccination, let alone to inform parents that their children risk death or permanent disability upon being vaccinated. I was equally dismayed to see first-hand the prevalence of physicians who are, if with the best of intentions, applying practices based on incomplete—and in some cases, outright mis—information.

This report is only a brief introduction; your own further investigation is warranted and strongly recommended. You may discover that this is the only way to get an objective view, as the controversy is a highly emotional one.

A word of caution: Many have found pediatricians unwilling or unable to discuss this subject calmly with an open mind. Perhaps this is because they have staked their personal identities and professional reputations on the presumed safety and effectiveness of vaccines, and because they are required by their profession to promote vaccination. But in any event, anecdotal reports suggest that most doctors have great difficulty acknowledging evidence of problems with vaccines. The first pediatrician I attempted to share my findings with yelled angrily at me when I calmly brought up the subject. The misconceptions have very deep roots.

Vaccination myth #1:

"Vaccines are safe . . . "
. . . or are they?

The Federal government VAERS (Vaccine Adverse Events Reporting System) was established by Congress under the National Childhood Vaccine Injury Compensation Act of 1986. It receives about 11,000 reports of serious adverse reactions to vaccinations annually, which include as many as one to two hundred deaths, and several times that number of permanent disabilities. VAERS officials report that 15% of adverse events are "serious" (emergency room trip, hospitalization, life-threatening episode, permanent disability, death). Independent analysis of VAERS reports has revealed that up to 50% of reported adverse events for the Hepatitis B vaccine are "serious." While these figures are alarming, they are only the tip of the iceberg. The FDA estimates that as few as 1% of serious adverse reactions to vaccines are reported, and the CDC admits that only about 10% of such events are reported. In fact, Congress has heard testimony that medical students are told not to report suspected adverse events.

The National Vaccine Information Center (NVIC, a grassroots organization founded by parents of vaccine-injured and killed children) has conducted its own investigations. It reported: "In New York, only one out of 40 doctor's offices confirmed that they report a death or injury following vaccination." In other words, 97.5% of vaccine related deaths and disabilities go unreported there. Implications about medical ethics aside (federal law directs doctors to report serious adverse events), these findings suggest that vaccine deaths and serious injuries actually occurring may be from 10 to 100 times greater than the number reported.

Researchers attribute dozens of chronic immunological and neurological diseases . . . to mass immunization campaigns.

With pertussis (often referred to as "whooping cough"), the number of vaccine-related deaths dwarfs the number of disease deaths, which have been about 10 annually for many years according to the CDC, and only 8 in 1993, one of the last peak-incidence years (pertussis runs in 3–4 year cycles; no one knows why, but vaccination rates have no such cycles). When you factor in under-reporting, the vaccine may be 100 times more deadly than the disease. Some argue that this is a necessary cost to prevent the return of a disease that would be more deadly than the vaccine. But when you consider the fact that the vast majority of disease decline in the twentieth century preceded the widespread use of vaccinations (pertussis mortality declined 79% prior to vaccines), and the fact that rates of disease declines remained virtually unchanged following the introduction of mass immunization, present day vaccine casualties cannot reasonably be explained away as a necessary sacrifice for the benefit of a disease-free society.

Unfortunately, the vaccine-related-deaths story doesn't end here.

Studies internationally have shown vaccination to be a cause of SIDS (SIDS, Sudden Infant Death Syndrome, is a "catch-all" diagnosis given when the specific cause of death is unknown; estimates range from 5,000 to 10,000 cases each year in the US). One study found the peak incidence of SIDS occurred at the ages of 2 and 4 months in the U.S., precisely when the first two routine immunizations are given, while another found a clear pattern of correlation extending three weeks after immunization. Another study found that 3,000 children die within 4 days of vaccination each year in the U.S. (amazingly, the authors reported no SIDS/vaccine relationship), while yet another researcher's studies led to the conclusion that at least half of SIDS cases are caused by vaccines.

Initial studies suggesting a causal relationship between SIDS and vaccines were quickly followed by vaccine-manufacturer-sponsored studies concluding that there is no relationship between SIDS and vaccines; one such study claimed that there was a slightly lower incidence of SIDS in vaccinees. However, many of these studies were called into question by yet another study that found "confounding" had erroneously skewed the results of these studies in favor of the vaccine. At best, there is conflicting evidence. But shouldn't we err on the side of caution? Shouldn't any credible correlation between vaccines and infant deaths be just cause for meticulous, widespread monitoring of the vaccination status of all SIDS cases? Health authorities have chosen to err on the side of denial rather than caution.

Present day vaccine casualties cannot reasonably be explained away as a necessary sacrifice for the benefit of a disease-free society.

In the mid 1970's Japan raised their vaccination age from two months to two years; their incidence of SIDS dropped dramatically; they went from an infant mortality ranking of 17 to first in the world (i.e., Japan had the lowest infant death rate when infants were not being immunized). England's vaccination rate temporarily dropped to about 30% at about the same time following media reports of vaccine-related brain damage. Infant mortality dropped substantially for about 2 years, then rose again in close correlation to rising immunization rates in the late 1970's. Despite these experiences, the medical community maintains a posture of denial. Coroners don't check the vaccination status of SIDS victims, and unsuspecting families continue to pay the price, unaware of the dangers and denied the right to make an informed choice.

FDA and CDC admissions about the lack of adverse event reporting suggests that the total number of adverse reactions actually occurring each year may actually fall within a range of 100,000 to a million (with "serious" events being approximately 20% of these). This concern is underscored by a study revealing that 1 in 175 children who completed the full DPT series suffered "severe reactions," and a Dr.'s report for attorneys stating that one in 300 DPT immunizations resulted in seizures.

England actually saw a drop in pertussis deaths when vaccination rates dropped to 30% in the mid 70's. Swedish epidemiologist B. Trollfors' study of pertussis vaccine efficacy and toxicity around the world found that "pertussis-associated mortality is currently very low in industrialised countries and no difference can be discerned when countries with high, low, and zero immunization rates were compared." He also found that England, Wales, and West Germany had more pertussis fatalities in 1970 when the immunization rate was high than during the last half of 1980, when rates had fallen.

Vaccinations cost us more than just the lives and health of our children. The U.S. Federal Government's National Vaccine Injury Compensation Program (NVICP) has paid out over $1.2 billion since 1988 to the families of children injured and killed by vaccines, with money that comes from a tax on vaccines that vaccine recipients pay. Meanwhile, pharmaceutical companies have a captive market; vaccines are legally mandated in all 50 U.S. states, yet these same companies are "immune" from accountability for the consequences of their products. Furthermore, they have been allowed to use "gag orders" as a leverage tool in vaccine damage legal settlements to prevent disclosure of information to the public about vaccination dangers. Such arrangements are clearly unethical; they force an uninformed American public to pay for vaccine manufacturer's liabilities, while ensuring that this same public will remain ignorant of the dangers of their products. This arrangement also diminishes any incentive that manufacturers might have to produce safer vaccines (after all, when the vaccine causes a death or injury, they don't have to pay for it; they still get their profit).

It is important to note that insurance companies, who do the best liability studies, refuse to cover vaccine reactions. Profits appear to dictate both the pharmaceutical and insurance companies' positions.

Vaccination truth #1:

"Vaccination causes significant death and disability at an astounding personal and financial cost to uninformed families."

Vaccination myth #2:

"Vaccines are very effective . . . "

. . . or are they?

The medical literature has a surprising number of studies documenting vaccine failure. Measles, mumps, smallpox, pertussis, polio and Hib (haemophilus influenzae type B) outbreaks have all occurred in vaccinated populations. In 1989 the CDC reported: "Among school-aged children, [measles] outbreaks have occurred in schools with vaccination levels of greater than 98 percent. [They] have occurred in all parts of the country, including areas that had not reported measles for years." The CDC even reported a measles outbreak in a documented 100% vaccinated population. A study examining this phenomenon concluded, *"The apparent paradox is that as measles immunization rates rise to high levels in a population, measles becomes a disease of immunized persons."* A more recent study found that measles vaccination *"produces immune suppression which contributes to an increased susceptibility to other infections."* These studies suggest that the goal of complete "immunization" may actually be counter-productive, a notion underscored by instances in which epidemics followed complete immunization of entire countries. Japan experienced yearly increases in smallpox following the introduction of compulsory vaccines in 1872. By 1892, there were 29,979 deaths, and all had been vaccinated. In the early 1900's, the Philippines experienced their worst smallpox epidemic ever after 8 million people received 24.5 million vaccine doses (achieving a vaccination rate of 95%); the death rate quadrupled as a result. Before England's first compulsory vaccination law in 1853, the largest two-year smallpox death rate was about 2,000; in 1870–71, England and Wales had over 23,000 smallpox deaths. In 1989, the country of Oman experienced a widespread polio outbreak six months after achieving complete vaccination. In the U.S. in 1986, 90% of 1300 pertussis cases in Kansas were *"adequately vaccinated."* 72% of pertussis cases in the 1993 Chicago outbreak were fully up to date with their vaccinations.

Vaccination truth #2:

"Evidence suggests that vaccination is an unreliable means of preventing disease."

Vaccination myth #3:

"Vaccines are the reason for low disease rates in the U.S. today . . . "

. . . *or are they?*

According to the British Association for the Advancement of Science, childhood diseases decreased 90% between 1850 and 1940, paralleling improved sanitation and hygienic practices, well before mandatory vaccination programs. The Medical Sentinel recently reported, "from 1911 to 1935, the four leading causes of childhood deaths from infectious diseases in the U.S. were diphtheria, pertussis, scarlet fever, and measles. However, by 1945 the combined death rates from these causes had declined by 95 percent, before the implementation of mass immunization programs."

Thus, at best, vaccinations can be examined only for their relationship to the small, remaining portion of disease declines that occurred after their introduction. Yet even this role is questionable, as pre-vaccine rates of disease mortality decline remained virtually the same after vaccines were introduced. Furthermore, European countries that refused immunization for smallpox and polio saw the epidemics end along with those countries that mandated it; vaccines were clearly not the sole determining factor. In fact, both smallpox and polio immunization campaigns were followed by significant disease incidence increases. After smallpox vaccination was being mandated, smallpox remained a prevalent disease with some substantial increases, while other infectious diseases simultaneously continued their declines in the absence of vaccines. In England and Wales, smallpox disease and vaccination rates eventually declined simultaneously over a period of several decades between the 1870's and the beginning of World War II. It is thus impossible to say whether or not vaccinations contributed to the continuing declines in disease death rates, or if the declines continued unabated simply due to the same forces which likely brought about the initial declines—improvements in sanitation, hygiene and diet; better housing, transportation and infrastructure; better food preservation techniques and technology; and natural disease cycles. Underscoring this conclusion was a recent World Health Organization report which found that the disease and mortality rates in third world countries have no direct correlation with immunization procedures or medical treatment, but are closely related to the standard of hygiene and diet. Credit given to vaccinations for our current disease incidence has simply been grossly exaggerated, if not outright misplaced.

Japan experienced yearly increases in smallpox following the introduction of compulsory vaccines in 1872.

Vaccine advocates point to incidence rather than mortality statistics as evidence of vaccine effectiveness. However, statisticians tell us that mortality statistics are a better measure of disease than incidence figures, for the simple reason that the quality of reporting and record keeping is much higher on fatalities. For instance, a survey in New York City revealed that only 3.2% of pediatricians were actually reporting measles cases to the health department. In 1974, the CDC determined that there were 36 cases of measles in Georgia, while the Georgia State Surveillance System reported 660 cases. In 1982, Maryland state health officials blamed a pertussis epidemic on a television program, "D.P.T.—Vaccine Roulette," which warned of the dangers of DPT; but when former top virologist for the U.S. Division of Biological Standards, Dr. J. Anthony Morris, analyzed the 41 cases, he confirmed only 5, and all had been vaccinated. Such instances as these demonstrate the fallacy of incidence figures, yet vaccine advocates tend to rely on them indiscriminately.

Vaccination truth #3

"It is unclear what impact, if any, that vaccines had on 19th and 20th century infectious disease declines."

Vaccination myth #4:

"Vaccination is based on sound immunization theory and practice . . . "
. . . *or is it?*

The clinical evidence for vaccines is their ability to stimulate antibody production in the recipient. What is not clear, however, is whether or not antibody production constitutes immunity. For example, agamma globulin-anemic children are incapable of producing antibodies, yet they recover from infectious diseases almost as quickly as other children. Furthermore, a study published by the British Medical Council in 1950 during a diphtheria epidemic concluded that there was no relationship between antibody count and disease incidence; researchers found resistant people with extremely low antibody counts and sick people with high counts. Natural immunization is a complex interactive process involving many bodily organs and systems; it cannot be replicated by the artificial stimulation of antibodies.

Research also indicates that vaccination commits immune cells to the specific antigens in a vaccine, rendering them incapable of reacting to other infections. Immunological reserves may thus actually be reduced, causing a generally lowered resistance.

Another component of immunization theory is "herd immunity," the notion that when enough people in a community are immunized, all are protected. As myth #2 showed, there are many documented instances showing just the opposite—fully vaccinated populations have experienced epidemics. With measles, this actually seems to be the direct result of high vaccination rates. In Minnesota, a state epidemiologist concluded that the Hib vaccine increases the risk of illness when a study revealed that vaccinated children were five times more likely to contract meningitis than unvaccinated children.

Surprisingly, vaccination has never actually been clinically proven to be effective in preventing disease, for the simple reason that no researcher has directly exposed test subjects to diseases (nor may they ethically do so). The medical community's gold standard, the double blind, placebo-controlled study, has not been used to compare vaccinated and unvaccinated people, and so the practice remains unscientifically proven. Furthermore, it is important to recognize that not everyone exposed to a disease develops symptoms (indeed, only a tiny percentage of a population need develop symptoms for an epidemic to be declared). Thus, if a vaccinated individual is exposed to a disease and doesn't get sick, it is impossible to know whether the vaccine worked, because there is no way to know if that person would have developed symptoms if he or she had not been vaccinated. It is also worth noting that outbreaks in recent years have recorded more disease cases in vaccinated children than in unvaccinated children.

Yet another surprising aspect of immunization practice is the "one size fits all" aspect. An 8 pound 2 month old baby receives the same dosage as a 40 pound five year old child. Infants with immature, undeveloped immune systems may receive five or more times the dosage, relative to body weight, as older children. Furthermore, the number of "units" within doses has been found in random testing to range from ½ to 3 times what the label indicates; manufacturing quality controls appear to tolerate a rather large margin of error. "Hot Lots"—vaccine lots associated with disproportionately high death and disability rates—have been repeatedly identified by the NVIC, but the FDA consistently refuses to intervene to prevent further unnecessary injury and deaths. In fact, individual vaccine lots have never been recalled due to their greater incidence of adverse reactions. However, the rotavirus vaccine was taken off the market a few months after being introduced when it caused bowel obstructions in many recipients. Incredibly, the FDA and CDC knew about this problem prior to licensing the vaccine, but both organizations still gave their unanimous approval.

Credit given to vaccinations for our current disease incidence has simply been grossly exaggerated.

Finally, vaccines are administered with the assumption that all recipients—regardless of race, culture, diet, genetic makeup, geographic location, or any other characteristic—will respond the same. This was perhaps never more dramatically disproved than in Australia's Northern Territory a few years ago, where stepped-up immunization campaigns in native aborigines resulted in an incredible 50% infant mortality rate. One must wonder about the lives of the survivors, too; if half died, surely the other half did not escape unaffected.

Almost as troubling was a recent study in the *New England Journal of Medicine* reporting that a substantial number of Romanian children were contracting polio from the vaccine. Researchers found a correlation with injections of antibiotics. A single injection within one month of vaccination raised the risk of polio eight times, two to nine injections raised the risk 27-fold, and 10 or more injections raised the risk 182 times.

Not only are most infectious diseases rarely dangerous, they can actually play a vital role in developing a strong, healthy immune system.

What other factors not accounted for in vaccination theory will surface unexpectedly to reveal unforeseen or previously overlooked consequences? We cannot begin to fully comprehend the scope and degree of the danger until public health officials begin looking and reporting in earnest. In the meantime, entire countries' populations are unwitting gamblers in a game that many might very well choose not to play if they were given all the rules in advance.

Vaccination truth #4:

"Many of the assumptions upon which immunization theory and practice are based are unproven or have been proven false in their application."

Vaccination myth #5:

"Childhood diseases are extremely dangerous . . . "

. . . *or are they, really?*

Most childhood infectious diseases have few serious consequences in today's modern world. Even conservative CDC statistics for pertussis during 1992–94 indicate a 99.8% recovery rate. In fact, when hundreds of pertussis cases occurred in Ohio and Chicago in the fall 1993 outbreak, an infectious disease expert from Cincinnati Children's Hospital said, *"The disease was very mild, no one died, and no one went to the intensive care unit."*

The vast majority of the time, childhood infectious diseases are benign and self-limiting. They usually impart lifelong immunity, whereas vaccine-induced immunity is only temporary. In fact, the temporary nature of vaccine immunity can create a more dangerous situation in a child's future. For example, the new chicken pox vaccine has an effectiveness estimated at 6 - 10 years. If effective, it will postpone the child's vulnerability until adulthood, when death from the disease, while still rare, is 20 times more likely than in childhood. "Measles parties" used to be common in Britain; if a child got measles, other parents in the neighborhood would rush their kids over to play with the infected child, to deliberately contract the disease and develop immunity. This avoids the risk of infection in adulthood when the disease is more dangerous, and provides the benefits of an immune system strengthened by the natural disease process.

About half of measles cases in the late 1980's resurgence were in adolescents and adults, most of whom were vaccinated as children, and the recommended booster shots may provide protection for less than six months. Some healthcare professionals are concerned that the virus from the chicken pox vaccine may *"reactivate later in life in the form of herpes zoster (shingles) or other immune system disorders."* Dr. A. Lavin of the Dept. of Pediatrics, St. Luke's Medical Center in Cleveland, Ohio, strongly opposed licensing the new vaccine, *"until we actually know . . . the risks involved in injecting mutated DNA [the vaccine herpes virus] into the host genome [children]."* The truth is, no one knows, but the vaccine is now licensed, recommended by health authorities, and quickly becoming mandated throughout the country.

Not only are most infectious diseases rarely dangerous, they can actually play a vital role in developing a strong, healthy immune system. Persons who have not had measles have a higher incidence of certain skin diseases, degenerative diseases of bone and cartilage, and certain tumors, while absence of mumps has been linked to higher risks of ovarian cancer. Anthroposophical medical doctors recommend only the tetanus and polio vaccines; they believe contracting the other childhood infectious diseases is beneficial in that it matures and strengthens the immune system.

Vaccination truth #5:

"Dangers of childhood diseases are greatly exaggerated in order to scare parents into compliance with a questionable but highly profitable procedure.". . .

Some closing remarks

In the December 1994 *Medical Post,* Canadian author of the best-seller *Medical Mafia,* Guylaine Lanctot, M.D., stated, "The medical authorities keep lying. Vaccination has been a disaster on the immune system. It actually causes a lot of illnesses. We are actually changing our genetic code through vaccination . . . 100 years from now we will know that the biggest crime against humanity was vaccines." After critically analyzing literally tens of thousands of pages of the vaccine medical literature, Dr. Viera Scheibner concluded that "there is no evidence whatsoever of the ability of vaccines to prevent any diseases. To the contrary, there is a great wealth of evidence that they cause serious side effects." Dr. Classen has stated, "My data proves that the studies used to support immunization are so flawed that it is impossible to say if immunization provides a net benefit to anyone or to society in general. This question can only be determined by proper studies which have never been performed. The flaw of previous studies is that there was no long-term follow up and chronic toxicity was not looked at. The American Society of Microbiology has promoted my research . . . and thus acknowledges the need for proper studies." To some these may seem like radical positions, but they are not unfounded. The continued denial and suppression of the evidence against vaccines only perpetuates the "myths" of their "success" and, more importantly, their negative consequences on our children and society. Aggressive and comprehensive scientific investigation into adverse vaccine events is clearly warranted, yet immunization programs continue to expand in the absence of such research. Manufacturer profits are enormous, while accountability for the negative effects is conspicuously absent. This is especially sad given the readily available safe and effective alternatives.

The positions asserted above are not coming from a handful of fringe lunatics; entire professional organizations are speaking out. Criticisms of vaccines are being sounded by an increasing number of credible and reputable scientists, researchers, investigators, and self-educated parents from around the world. Instead, it is public health officials and die-hard vaccine advocates (many of whom have a financial stake in the outcome of the debate) who are beginning to lose credibility by refusing to acknowledge the growing body of evidence and to address the very real, serious, documented problems.

Meanwhile, the race is on. There are over 200 new vaccines being developed for everything from birth control to cocaine addiction. Some 100 of these are already in clinical trials. Researchers are working on vaccine delivery through nasal sprays, mosquitoes (yes, mosquitoes), and the fruits of "transgenic" plants in which vaccine viruses are grown. With every adult and child on the planet a potential recipient of vaccines administered periodically throughout their lives, and every healthcare system and government a potential buyer, it is little wonder that countless millions of dollars are spent nurturing the growing multi-billion dollar vaccine industry. Without public outcry, we will see more and more new vaccines required of us all. And while profits are readily calculable, the real human costs are ignored or suppressed.

Whatever your personal vaccination decision, make it an informed one; you have that right and responsibility. It is a difficult issue, but there is more than enough at stake to justify whatever time and energy it takes.

4

Vaccine Shortages Threaten Public Health

Sarah Wildman

Sarah Wildman is an assistant editor for the New Republic.

The United States is currently undergoing shortages of several vaccines that are required by law for children. These shortages place the population at risk because underimmunized children could catch and spread diseases that can lead to dangerous illness-related complications in adults and pregnant women. Today's shortages are largely the result of economic disincentives: The pharmaceutical industry does not profit much from vaccine production, and a number of companies have stopped making vaccines in the wake of several immunization-related lawsuits. To alleviate the dangers posed by vaccine shortages, some analysts have suggested creating a National Vaccine Authority, an alliance between government and private industry that would oversee immunizations in the United States.

A child is sick: high fever, acutely sensitive to light, spots break out all over her body. Another child falls ill. Suddenly hundreds are infected and dozens are hospitalized. Deaths are feared. Smallpox? Anthrax? A terrorist attack? Try measles—in Germany—in March 2002. The same thing happened one decade ago in the United States: 11,000 were hospitalized and 123 died.

It could easily happen again. And not just with measles. Currently the United States is experiencing shortages of eight of the eleven vaccines required by law for children: measles, mumps, rubella, diphtheria, tetanus, pertussis (whooping cough), varicella (chicken pox), and pneumococcal disease (meningitis). In response, the Centers for Disease Control (CDC) have revised their immunization schedule from "optimal" to "some protection," which means that, depending on the vaccine, kids may get the first shot and not the boosters that solidify immunity, or they may not get the first shot at all until several months past the recommended age. In response to the shortages, some states are relaxing their demands that kids get vaccinated before they come to school in September 2002. In Oregon, for example, seven-year-olds will be allowed to forgo chicken pox shots and diphtheria/tetanus boosters; Texas is deferring the diphtheria/tetanus booster shot required for all 14-year-olds. Which is scary, because children aren't the only ones at risk: Spotty vaccination cycles for diseases such as rubella and chicken pox mean that children may grow to adulthood without immunity, remaining at risk for diseases that cause many more complications for adults and can have devastating effects for pregnant women.

The pharmaceutical industry and the CDC promise to alleviate the shortages by the end of 2002. But America's national vaccine supply is so "fragile"—according to several prominent immunologists—that, even if they do, shortages will almost surely return. "These shortages speak to a bigger problem, which is that at some level there is a slight crumbling of infrastructure," warns Dr. Paul Offit, an infectious disease expert at Children's Hospital of Philadelphia. "It's only going to get worse." Which is why the terrorism-addled federal government, which in 2002 plans to spend $640 million to build stockpiles of the vaccine for smallpox—a disease that hasn't killed anyone in 25 years—needs to start worrying about something more mundane and perhaps more dangerous: a deadly outbreak of measles.

Most people assume the diseases that ravaged millions in the early twentieth century no longer affect American children. And in good years, when American kids get their required vaccines on schedule, that's true. In the 1950s nearly every American child came down with measles by the time he or she was seven, and the number of measles cases hovered around four million per year. But with the introduction of a measles vaccine in 1963, that number plummeted to a few hundred cases per year. The same is true for diphtheria, a disease that claimed more than 15,000 lives annually before a vaccine was instituted in 1923; today it's all but eradicated in the United States.

America's national vaccine supply is so "fragile". . . [that] shortages will almost surely return.

But not every country is so lucky. In Russia, for instance, a mid-1990s diphtheria outbreak infected 80,000 people and left 2,000 dead. And people from Russia, Germany, China, Britain, and other countries where vaccination is less routine enter the United States in large numbers every day. When the United States keeps its vaccine levels above roughly 90 percent, according to immunologists, that's not a big problem because of "herd immunity." Thanks to herd immunity, immigrants who aren't vaccinated—or for that matter native-born Americans who aren't vaccinated—ride on the backs of the rest of the population and are protected. A child or adult who is ill arrives in Seattle, walks into a Starbucks, a grocery store, a movie theater. But because pretty much everyone in those public spaces has been vaccinated, the disease runs its course through that one person, infecting perhaps the one other nonimmunized person the carrier comes across, rather than being passed on to nearly everyone

he meets. The key is keeping vaccine levels up: If they fall below 90 percent, preventable diseases begin finding the chinks in our immunization
armor and sweeping through the population. America's early '90s measles
outbreak, for instance, started among undocumented immigrant children
in Texas and California and the urban poor in Philadelphia and
Chicago—where large numbers of children were undervaccinated or not
vaccinated at all. But it quickly spread beyond those populations, affect-
ing even children in states with higher vaccination levels.

The cause of vaccine shortages

So what's causing the vaccine shortages that threaten our herd immunity
today? The answer begins and ends with our peculiar quasi-free-market
approach to producing vaccines. Though undoubtedly a public utility,
vaccines are manufactured exclusively by independent pharmaceutical
companies. This isn't in and of itself a bad thing: Private sector indepen-
dence often breeds innovation. The problem is that the incentive for such
innovation is profit. And unlike blockbuster drugs that lower cholesterol
or reduce anxiety, vaccines are notoriously unprofitable.

For one thing, they are difficult to create: They often require handling
live viruses, and some take nearly one year to produce. What's more, the
Food and Drug Administration (FDA) has recently clamped down on the
manufacture of vaccines, requiring pharmaceutical companies to make
multimillion-dollar quality-control upgrades to their production facilities
in order to comply with what's called "good manufacturing practice" and
to ensure uniform safety standards. The FDA also recently decided that
vaccines could no longer be preserved in a solution called thimerosal, a
mercury-based concoction long used in multidose vials of certain vaccines. Companies whose vaccines were sitting in thimerosal had to switch
from multi- to single-dose vials—a transfer that immediately reduced supplies by 25 percent—as single-dose vials must be overfilled to allow sy-
ringes to withdraw the appropriate amount.

And once the vaccines get to market, they don't fetch top dollar.
Some 50 percent to 60 percent of vaccines are bought by the government,
which typically purchases them at near cost. "The trend [is] to shoot for
the lowest possible price whenever there's a negotiation between government—which is the country's largest purchaser—and the industry," says
Dr. Tom Zink, a representative of pharma giant GlaxoSmithKline. The
other 40 percent of the vaccine market—covered primarily by private-
sector health insurance and out of pocket by the underinsured—doesn't
help much either because Americans, most of whom don't remember the
tragedy of diseases like diphtheria, generally chafe at paying high costs
for vaccines. As Offit notes, many people balk at spending $10 for an in-
fluenza vaccine, though it would cost more than ten times that amount
to treat the illness itself. And even for those vaccines that do cost more—
like the new meningitis vaccine, which costs $250 for a live-course dose—
the cost is only paid once per patient. Compare that to pricey drugs like
cholesterol-lowering Lipitor that are taken daily for years.

As a result of these economic disincentives (combined with various
lawsuits that scared off several pharmaceutical-industry players), over the
last 20 years the number of companies producing vaccines has dropped

from 15 to four. And there is little overlap in production between the remaining four, which means stockpiles are often minimal or nonexistent. In December 2001, for instance, a company called Wyeth Lederle decided to stop producing the DTaP (diphtheria/tetanus/pertussis) vaccine with only one month's notice. That left Aventis Pasteur as the only company still marketing the tetanus vaccine in the United States. And Aventis didn't have enough supply to make up for the loss. The result was, and remains, that the tetanus vaccine is unavailable almost anywhere in the country except emergency rooms.

If [vaccination levels] fall below 90 percent, preventable diseases begin finding the chinks in our immunization armor and sweeping through the population.

The irony, as Dr. Louis Cooper, president of the American Academy of Pediatrics, points out, is that "immunizations are the most cost-beneficial medical invention in history." Next to purifying the water supply, nothing has been as "profoundly effective" in improving public health at such a low cost. "What we have to do," says Cooper, "is take a step back and look at how we align incentives. . . . Because drug companies are not philanthropies. If you were a CEO of a drug company and you looked at your portfolio, do you invest in a vaccine or a hypertensive or an anti-anxiety or anti-pain medication? Where is the return on investment quicker and profoundly more?"

Creating a National Vaccine Authority

One option—proposed by the Institute of Medicine (IOM), a nonprofit research arm of the National Academy of Sciences—is a National Vaccine Authority (NVA), a public-private partnership charged with overseeing immunizations across the country. With the NVA, says IOM president Dr. Kenneth Shine, "government involvement would only occur when the market is not meeting demands." He suggests the creation of a government-owned facility or a contract between private industry and the government, like the one the Department of Defense has set up to create vaccines for bioterrorism.

Industry, not surprisingly, balks at establishing another bureaucratic agency. And not without reason. In fact, something like the NVA already exists; it's called the National Vaccine Program (NVP), a congressionally mandated bureaucracy set up to coordinate the efforts of various federal agencies involved in vaccinations. Rather than starting from scratch, the NVP could be significantly strengthened. An important first step would simply be improving the currently poor state of communication between the various agencies and corporations that comprise the NVP. "Close, tight communication between industry, the Department of Health and Human Services, the CDC, [and] the FDA on issues relating to vaccines" is imperative, says Lance Rodewald, director of the Immunization Services Division at the CDC. Manufacturers, suggests Rodewald, might be required to notify the government further in advance when they plan to stop making vaccines so other companies have time to ramp up production.

A stronger NVP could also press the FDA to work with international drug manufacturers in an effort to "harmonize requirements across countries." If production standards were harmonized across borders, the United States could import vaccines to alleviate supply shortages, which it can't easily do today. The NVP could also do a better job of tracking current stockpiles and encouraging the creation of additional stores. Because many vaccines expire if left to sit like computer paper on a shelf, they must be cycled through and distributed to keep the stash on hand as fresh as possible. The NVP could make sure that both manufacturers and the federal government keep their supplies current and plentiful.

Of course, all this will take more money from Congress. And so far Congress hasn't been particularly interested in handing it over. In the year 2000 the Institute of Medicine recommended $75 million in additional funding for the NVP; but Congress appropriated only $42.5 million. Fortunately, the General Accounting Office is due to issue a report at the end of July 2002 examining the vaccine shortages, which will hopefully prompt Congress to take the issue more seriously.

But in the meantime, children across the country are being sent home from their pediatricians without the shots they require. "[A]ny underimmunized child anywhere in the country puts the rest of the country at risk," Dr. Walter Orenstein, director of the National Immunization Program at the CDC, has said. The more kids don't get their immunizations, the more likely long-forgotten diseases like measles will return to afflict Americans. Which would be shameful, because this form of bioterrorism is entirely preventable.

5

Contaminated Vaccines Threaten Public Health

Leonard G. Horowitz, interviewed by Roger G. Mazlen

Independent investigator Leonard G. Horowitz is the author of Emerging Viruses: AIDS and Ebola—Nature, Accident, or Intentional? *Roger G. Mazlen is the former host of the* Chronic Fatigue Syndrome Radio Show.

The current proliferation of unusual cancers and autoimmune illnesses is the result of large populations being inoculated with vaccines that are known to be contaminated. For example, the oral polio vaccine (OPV) is prepared in monkey kidney tissues that often contain contaminants such as herpes, the Epstein-Barr virus, and other immune-suppressing agents. This vaccine has been given to more than 100 million people around the world. Moreover, twentieth-century research into developing biological weapons and anticancer vaccines—which entailed recombining various animal viruses—may have resulted in AIDS and AIDS-related illnesses. The Food and Drug Administration does not share this information with the public due to binding nondisclosure agreements it has with the pharmaceutical industry.

Editor's Note: This viewpoint is a transcript of an interview that originally aired on the Chronic Fatigue Syndrome Radio Show *on March 15, 1998.*

*R*oger G. Mazlen: We have as our guest Dr Leonard Horowitz, a Harvard graduate, independent investigator and internationally known authority on public health education, who's the author of the best-selling book Emerging Viruses: AIDS and Ebola.
Why are we talking to Dr Horowitz? Simply, chronic fatigue syndrome (CFS) patients have a depressed immune system. They have immune deficiency. They have immune suppression. They are sitting ducks for any kind of new viruses, especially those with the ability to destroy the immune system. So, without any further ado, welcome to the show, Dr Horowitz.

From "Vaccine Contamination: Germ Warfare on Civilians?" by Leonard G. Horowitz and Roger G. Mazlen, *NEXUS*, June/July 1998. Copyright © 1998 by Leonard G. Horowitz. Reprinted with permission.

Leonard G. Horowitz: Thank you, Dr Mazlen. It's a great privilege and pleasure to be with you.

Well, we're delighted that we're able to talk to you today. Let me let you start by introducing us to the general scope of your book.

Well, I spent three years investigating a 1970 Department of Defense appropriations request for $10 million into a five-year study to develop immune-system-ravaging micro-organisms for germ warfare. I didn't believe at first that this was a legitimate document. Ultimately I tracked the money following a paper trail of scientific literature and government documents and I found that the money had gone to an organisation called Litton Bionetics. Did you ever hear of Litton microwave ovens?

Surely.

Well, they're also a subsidiary of a megamilitary weapons contracting firm and they had a medical subsidiary which was called Litton Bionetics. They were sixth on the list with major army biological weapons contractors during the late '60s and early '70s. And they commuted numerous immune-system-ravaging micro-organisms for germ warfare. They were the recipients of over $2 million a year to develop these types of micro-organisms, not only for biological weapons research and development but also for cancer research and vaccine research and development. So, that's basically the book. *Emerging Viruses: AIDS and Ebola* goes into who made these types of viruses—the AIDS-like, Ebola-like viruses—how they made them, virtually every step of the way, and why they made them. And then, most incredibly, I found and reprinted in black and white the US Government contracts which show you how much US taxpayers pay to finance these research efforts.

Contaminated vaccines

Well, of course, this is a very serious concern to our listening audience—those who have chronic fatigue, or those who suspect they may have, or those who are not sure—because any new virus or any virus which has the ability to suppress immunity constitutes a major threat to these people and to the general public as well.

Now, in your book, and I'm going to quote you, on page 134 you say: "Putting all the facts together I now understood how humanly benign DNA monkey viruses, like SV40. . .and other common retrovirus vaccine contaminants like SFV, could have, over the period of a few decades, become RNA retroviruses that, through contaminated vaccines, spread to millions of people around the world." Could you amplify that a little bit for the audience?

Certainly. The gist of the book and the warning of the book *Emerging Viruses: AIDS and Ebola* is that we have a Food and Drug Administration [FDA] that does not tell health scientists or health professionals or the public the truth about the contaminated vaccines or the methods by which the vaccines are prepared. For example, the oral polio vaccine is still, to this day, being prepared in contaminated monkey kidney tissues which are bringing with it a variety of not only monkey virus contaminants but also the herpes-type viruses, such as simian cytomegalovirus, Epstein-Barr and herpes B, which we know are immune-system-suppressing types of viruses.

We know also that the vaccine that most plausibly delivered AIDS and possibly even chronic fatigue to the world—since they both broke out in the same year, 1978—was the 1974 experimental hepatitis B vaccine that was prepared in Merck, Sharpe & Dohme's laboratories, along with support from the Centers for Disease Control and the Food and Drug Administration. We know that this particular hepatitis B vaccine was partly prepared in contaminated monkeys that were shipped by Litton—again, a biological weapons contracting firm for the Department of Defense. And we know for a fact that the monkeys from which these vaccines were produced were contaminated. We even have testimonial by the man who created these vaccines to that effect. His name is Dr Maurice Hilleman, and he was Merck, Sharpe & Dohme's leading vaccine developer.

We have a Food and Drug Administration that does not tell health scientists or health professionals or the public the truth about . . . contaminated vaccines.

So they developed these vaccines partly in contaminated animals and then they inoculated them into human beings, and it was therefore an accident waiting to happen that we would have a variety of immune-system-related disorders including weird cancers and weird auto-immune illnesses that we have in epidemic proportions today.

Well that, of course, brings up a lot of issues, but I want to go back to your book again where you quote an interview with Dr Hilleman by Edward Shorter, PhD [pages 484–5], where Hilleman said, "there were 40 different viruses in these vaccines anyway that we were inactivating", and Shorter responded, "But you weren't inactivating the [SV40, simian virus 40]. . ." And then Hilleman said, "No, that's right." And he even went on to say, "But yellow fever vaccine had leukaemia virus in it, and you know this is in the days of very crude science."

So, here we now learn from the very statements they made that not only were there immune-damaging viruses, there were even viruses that could spread leukaemia virus. You do go into this in the book. You talk about cases of T-cell leukaemia. What about that, for example? Is there still some risk of that occurring?

I believe so, Dr Mazlen. I believe that many of these risks still continue to this day. Let me give you an example. Today, the Food and Drug Administration, which we rely upon for both our personal and our children's health and safety, must turn a blind eye to as many as 100 monkey virus contaminants per dose of the oral polio vaccine that we're allegedly by law told we must give our children today. And I say "allegedly" because it's not true. We have spiritual and religious exemptions that you can get, and it is actually voluntary, but they make it seem like you can't go to school or you can't get your children into schools or you can't work in, for example, healthcare settings without getting these vaccines—and that's not the truth.

But you see, the Food and Drug Administration must turn a blind eye to at least 100 of these contaminants per dose because their hands are tied by proprietary laws and non-disclosure agreements placed upon them by the pharmaceutical industry. In other words, they're muzzled by the drug makers. So they can't even tell our scientists the true extent of the contaminations and the risks associated with the vaccines. Therefore, the physicians—who get most of their continuing medical education paid for by the pharmaceutical industry as well—never learn the truth; and subsequently, when they look at patients with running eyes and say that these vaccines are "for your own good" or "for your children's own good", they believe it. And they're just basically brainwashed. They're like cult followers, but they don't even know who their cult leaders are in many cases.

Well, we certainly don't get any real information on the process of vaccine-making in medical school. I mean, there really isn't anything in the curriculum. I don't remember anything in the curriculum that applies to that whatsoever; and so, as you say, it's a fait accompli. *You are just told to do it. It's good and you do it. This changes the whole picture, because in good conscience you wouldn't be giving something if you knew that it was contaminated with something that's detrimental.*

A stealth virus

Now we're going to talk a little bit about the work that's been done by W. John Martin and how it fits into this book. Dr W. John Martin, MD, PhD, wrote the foreword to this book and there's a section in it in which Dr Horowitz talks about Martin's experience at the FDA at a time when he was director of the Viral Oncology Branch at the FDA's Bureau of Biologics [now the Center for Biologics, Evaluation and Research] and that he had been informed that there was contamination by simian cytomegalovirus. This is important because Dr Martin has been reporting cases of a stealth virus—a CMV virus, which is in the herpes family—in the Mohave Valley area in Arizona, which has been spreading in every direction and toward the major cities and population centres. I would like it very much if you would comment on this.

The [FDA] must turn a blind eye to . . . these contaminants . . . because their hands are tied by proprietary laws and non-disclosure agreements placed upon them by the pharmaceutical industry.

Sure, Dr Mazlen, I'd be happy to. Now this basically comes from personal conversations with Dr Martin. Dr Martin, of course, as you mentioned, wrote the foreword to this book, *Emerging Viruses,* and he talks about his experience as the Bureau of Biologics vaccine tester and actually in charge of testing humans for vaccine contamination between 1976 and 1980. At one point in the book he cites the fact that there's no reason for these vaccines to continue to be contaminated, that the authorities hold the capacity and the technology to clean them up but yet they don't. Well, I go into detail about the social-political background on that, and I'm not going to go into that on your program today because we don't have the time, but let me give you one example.

When Dr Martin found some of these foreign viruses, DNA viruses and RNA viruses in the vaccines, he went to his superior at the FDA bureau and said to him: "You know, we've got a problem with these vaccines." And his boss said to him: "Stop worrying about it. Every time you eat an apple, you ingest foreign DNA." That was the response.

Today . . . we're still getting and we're still giving contaminated monkey viruses to human beings.

That's not too comforting, overall. In fact, it's a comment that leads one to feel a certain sense of insecurity about vaccines, and there have been times when we've had guests on this program who commented about whether or not they should give vaccines to their children or to people with chronic fatigue syndrome. It makes it difficult to counsel them because you're really not sure what's there. Now specifically, Martin also mentions—and you say it in the book—that the SV40 which was in the oral polio vaccines is actually pretty much carried in the general community and it's spreading.

Right, and as a matter of fact it was, I think, three weeks ago [in February 1998] now when the *Journal of the American Medical Association [JAMA]* carried the first article showing that the simian virus 40, the 40th monkey virus ever discovered, was known in 1961 to be contaminating both Salk and Sabin polio vaccines and that, in fact, those vaccines had been given to well over 100 million people around the world, mostly in Russia.

According to Hilleman—we have him on tape, again being interviewed by Shorter—the joke of the day in 1961 became, since they had just inoculated mostly Russians with this contaminated vaccine, that the Russian athletes were going to come to the next Olympics full of tumours.

Well, you see, they never cleaned them up, not completely; and today, again, we're still getting and we're still giving contaminated monkey viruses to human beings.

The article in *JAMA* discusses specific types of cancers—"unique cancers", they said—and states that the general public should not be concerned. And I beg to differ with them. I think it should be an extreme concern. I think we should literally have a moratorium on US Government–promulgated vaccines until there is a thorough, independent scientific investigation as well as, hopefully, a congressional investigation into all the documented facts. But the *JAMA* article said that there were now *unique* cancers associated with SV40.

An earlier article talked about 25 per cent of a very large Italian population carrying these monkey viruses in their bodies, and I suspect that it's a larger percentage here in the United States.

Cancer-ridden vaccines

A woman by the name of Bernice Eddy [a doctor of bacteriology] discovered [in 1954, with cancer researcher Sarah Stewart] this particular virus that was first called SE polyoma. She discovered this virus in contaminated polio vaccines, and she took photographs of a dozen monkeys which had keeled over dead and paralyzed when she administered the vaccine. Her boss at the National Institutes of Health (NIH) confiscated the photos and demoted and defunded her; and then 10 years of crusading later, in 1972, she gets before Congress and she tells the United States Congress people: "If you continue to allow these contaminated vaccines to go out, I guarantee you that over the next 20 years you will have epidemics of cancer unlike the world has ever seen." And that's precisely what we have today.

Certainly, if you include the AIDS virus as part of this, no doubt. In terms of your research—which is extensive in the book, and I certainly think that anyone who reads it will be impressed by the amount of work you've done—you do go into, at length, the fact that the AIDS virus might have come about through synthetic development, blending a number of killer viruses in an effort to make an immune-destroying virus. When did that happen?

This type of research, wherein simian virus 40 and other monkey viruses were used and then mutated or hybridised with other animal cancer viruses, began in the early 1960s. The contracts that are reprinted in *Emerging Viruses* show that it was February 12, 1962 that the Special Virus Cancer Program began. That was a largely funded, mostly secret program that resulted after the people on the inside at the National Institutes of Health realised they had just inoculated well over 100 million people around the world with cancer-virus-ridden vaccines.

When they started this, it was kind of like the ground floor of a huge business opportunity at that point, and they began to do extensive research in mutating monkey viruses to see what would produce cancer with them, and then, perhaps, how they might be treated with vaccines and whatever else.

So, it was in the '60s, and particularly by the late '60s, that researchers at Litton Bionetics—Dr Robert Gallo was overseeing them—and researchers at the National Cancer Institute as well, were very adept at taking monkey viruses and recombining them with things like feline leukaemia virus RNA that caused a whole laundry list of symptoms virtually identical to what AIDS patients suffer from. Another favourite one that they used to mutate monkey viruses with, was the chicken leukaemia sarcoma virus RNA that caused wasting, immunosuppression and death. And then the researchers recorded that to get this type of a virus to jump species readily—they cultured it in human white blood cells in some studies and human foetal tissue cells in culture in other studies so that it would adapt—the virus would develop what's called the "attachment apparatus". Those are the unique proteins like the gp 120-like protein.

A couple of very important things I want to say before we have to close the show for today. One, is it safe for people to donate blood if you're not screening for SV40 and simian CMV virus?

No, I think not. I think that's a very urgent question that should also be addressed by independent scientific investigation and congressional investigation. You see, the blood bankers—the international blood "banksters", as I like to call them—are the people who allowed 10,000 haemophiliacs throughout the United States to get HIV-contaminated blood. And recently we've been told that if you had a blood transfusion between 1970 and 1990, you'd better go get checked for the cancer ticking-time-bomb virus called hepatitis C. These are the same people who have allowed these types of things. They're very related financially and otherwise to the companies that have been producing the contaminated vaccines. And my concern is that they're making vast fortunes off humanity's suffering through the healthcare system; and people are dying off on this planet. It's interesting that that fulfils a very clear and well-articulated, well-documented population reduction agenda. So I'm concerned about those issues.

We're going to have you back at another time to talk about some of this. Because there's going to be a lot of people who are interested in your book and your research, what number can they reach you at about these things?

Well, the materials can be gained by calling a toll-free number [in the USA]. It's 1888 508 4787. An easy way to remember that number is 1888-50-VIRUS. And I'm pleased to tell you that despite the fact that, [during 1997 and 1998], all the major chain-store buyers have refused to buy the book—in other words, there has been a boycott against the book, *Emerging Viruses: AIDS and Ebola*—it did become a best seller in hardcover [in December 1997].

Congratulations on that. I want to ask you, though, are you researching now what's happening with some of these things? The hepatitis B vaccine you implicated might have been contaminated at one point in time. Is it still contaminated?

Yes, it is. As a matter of fact, I came back from France not too long ago, where I met with one of the top virologists in the world—a cancer virologist who used to work with Gallo and Montagnier. His name is Merko Valjenski, and he basically gave me some scientific documents showing that today's hepatitis B vaccine is still carrying a very carcinogenic enzyme that the authorities have not yet removed.

6

Currently Available Vaccines Are Not Contaminated

Centers for Disease Control and Prevention

The Centers for Disease Control and Prevention (CDC) is a federal government agency that is charged with tracking disease and assisting state public health agencies.

Today's vaccines do not contain contaminants that can cause disease, as a few researchers have claimed. For example, no reliable evidence has confirmed allegations that polio vaccine is contaminated by a so-called "stealth" virus. While simian virus 40 (SV 40) was found in some lots of polio vaccine in the early 1960s, there is no evidence that it causes cancer or other illnesses in humans, and today's vaccine manufacturers are required to test their products for SV 40. The Food and Drug Administration ensures that careful clinical trials are conducted on all vaccines before they are approved for distribution in the United States.

There is no reliable evidence that currently available vaccines are contaminated with infectious agents that cause disease. Today, manufacturers are required to test cell lines used in the production of vaccines for the presence of a variety of infectious agents, to prevent contamination of vaccine products. The following issues have been proposed by some as potential infectious agents: reverse transcriptase (RT), a "stealth" virus, simian virus 40 (SV40), and fetal tissue.

Reverse transcriptase

Vaccines produced using chick embryo may contain minute quantities of an avian enzyme necessary for a retrovirus to reproduce. This enzyme does not confirm the presence of a retrovirus. In addition, this enzyme is not derived from the human immunodeficiency virus (HIV), a well-known retrovirus.

Reverse transcriptase (RT) is an enzyme necessary for retroviruses to reproduce. Retroviruses are found in many different species. RT is not in-

From "Concerns About Vaccine Contamination," by Centers for Disease Control and Prevention, www.cdc.gov, September 28, 1997.

fectious in humans or animals, and it has not been shown to cause any adverse health effects in people. Using a highly sensitive polymerase chain reaction (PCR) based assay, RT activity has been detected in minute quantities in vaccines manufactured with chick embryo fibroblasts. The source of the enzyme is probably a partial viral genome coding for RT, believed to be integrated into chick cells hundreds or thousands of years ago. Avian retroviruses that produce this RT are not known to affect humans. While the human immunodeficiency virus (HIV, the virus that leads to AIDS), is a retrovirus, the RT activity detected in vaccines is definitively not derived from HIV. Furthermore, the presence of RT does not confirm the presence of a retrovirus.

Among vaccines with evidence of RT are the measles, mumps, influenza, and yellow fever vaccines. The presence of RT does not necessarily indicate the presence of a retrovirus that could cause infection or lead to illness in humans. In fact, investigations of the vaccines and the chick cells from which they were produced, conducted by the Centers for Disease Control and Prevention (CDC), the Food and Drug Administration (FDA), and others, have found no evidence of an infectious, transmissible retrovirus.

"Stealth" virus

There is no evidence that polio vaccine, or any other vaccine, has been contaminated with a "stealth" virus. To our knowledge, existence of this virus as suggested by one researcher has not been confirmed by other investigators.

"Stealth" virus is the label that one researcher has given to a cytopathic virus he has described. He has suggested that such viruses may reside within the body without being detected by the immune system. There is no evidence that polio vaccine, or any other vaccine, has been contaminated with a "stealth" virus. To our knowledge, existence of this virus has not been confirmed by other investigators.

There is no reliable evidence that currently available vaccines are contaminated with infectious agents that cause disease.

The researcher reports that the "stealth" virus or a related virus has been cultured from the tissues of patients with chronic fatigue syndrome and other chronic neuropsychiatric and autoimmune conditions. He further suggests that the "stealth" virus could be the cause of these illnesses. These findings have not been confirmed by any other investigators. Moreover, it has been stated that the same researcher found similar rates of viral detection among persons with chronic fatigue syndrome and control persons without these illnesses in a blinded study. If a "stealth" virus were a cause of these illnesses, higher rates of infection would be expected among ill persons, compared with healthy control subjects.

He has reported that a partial sequence of this virus is like that of simian cytomegalovirus (SCMV) and suggests that the source of the

SCMV-like virus is the African Green monkey. Because African Green monkey kidney cells are used in production of live oral polio vaccine, he hypothesized that the SCMV-like virus ("stealth" virus) may be an adventitious agent in polio vaccines. The researcher's results have not been confirmed in independent laboratories (the usual way to confirm scientific findings) to date.

There is no evidence that polio vaccine, or any other vaccine, has been contaminated with a "stealth" virus.

At a workshop in July 1996, the FDA and National Institutes of Health scientists reviewed some of this scientist's observations. The results presented were considered inconclusive. The need for sharing among scientists of methods and reagents was emphasized so that other workers might independently evaluate the methods and conclusions. The FDA considers that the methods applied by the manufacturer to test for SCMV in polio vaccine would detect replicating SCMV.

Simian virus 40

This virus has no relationship to HIV or simian immunodeficiency virus (SIV). In the early 1960s, some lots of polio vaccines were discovered to contain SV40. Since 1961, manufacturers have been required by the Food and Drug Administration to test for SV40. There is limited evidence that SV40 can infect humans, but there is no evidence it causes human health problems.

Simian virus 40 was discovered in the early 1960s to be present in some lots of polio vaccines. It was found in the inactivated (injectable) polio vaccine and some experimental lots of oral polio vaccine. The polio vaccine in those lots had been manufactured in kidney cells from simians (monkeys) that harbored SV40. The control methods used before this time did not identify this adventitious agent. The formalin inactivation process used to kill the poliovirus was found not to inactivate the SV40 completely. Beginning in 1961, manufacturers have been required by FDA to test for SV40, using modified methods and different cell cultures, and lots positive for SV40 are not released. A few years later, the source of monkeys used for production was changed to species that do not harbor SV40.

SV40 is a polyomavirus. It has no relationship to HIV or simian immunodeficiency virus (SIV; the virus that causes AIDS in monkeys). SV40 can cause cancer in laboratory animals. Limited evidence suggests that SV40 can infect humans, but there is no evidence that it causes human health problems. Recent publications have identified SV40 DNA sequences in samples of tissue from rare human tumors, including choroid plexus tumors, mesotheliomas, ependymomas, and osteosarcomas, as well as in apparently normal (non-neoplastic) human tissue. However, this finding has not been confirmed by some investigators. The entire SV40 genome has been isolated from one human choroid plexus tumor.

People who received polio vaccine between 1954 and 1962 may have received a dose that contained SV40. As many as 10 to 30 million persons in the U.S. could have received SV40-contaminated injectable polio vaccine. The participants of several clinical trials (approximately 10,000 persons) may have received oral polio vaccine that was contaminated with SV40. Studies in the U.S. have shown no increased rates of cancer among persons who would have received polio vaccine between 1954 and 1962; similarly, studies in Sweden have not shown any increased risk for cancers among people exposed to vaccines potentially containing SV40, compared with people who were not exposed to these vaccines. Moreover, there is no evidence that polio vaccine administered since the early 1960s contained SV40. For decades, manufacturers have been required by FDA to test for SV40 using infectivity assays.

Fetal tissue and vaccines

No new fetal tissue is used to produce vaccines. Cell lines generated from a single fetal tissue source are sometimes used for some vaccines. Vaccine manufacturers obtain human cell lines from FDA-certified cell banks.

Some vaccines such as rubella and varicella are made from human cell-line cultures, and some of these cell lines originated from aborted fetal tissue, obtained from legal abortions in the 1960s. No new fetal tissue is needed to produce cell lines to make these vaccines, now or in the future.

In 1964, there were an estimated 20,000 babies born with congenital rubella syndrome (CRS) in the United States. When women contract rubella disease during early pregnancy, this often causes miscarriage or neurological damage to the unborn child, resulting in the child suffering blindness, deafness and retardation. In 1993, the number of CRS cases was seven, reflecting a 99.9% reduction in this preventable disease since 1964.

In 1996, CDC, the American Academy of Pediatrics and the American Academy of Family Physicians jointly recommended routine use of varicella vaccine to protect children from chickenpox. In March 1995, this vaccine was licensed for use in the United States by the FDA and was shown to be safe and effective. Widespread use of varicella vaccine—which took more than 20 years for development, testing, and licensing—can help prevent thousands of children from being hospitalized each year because of complications from chickenpox. Complications of chickenpox include secondary infections such as group A streptococcal infections, which can lead to necrotizing fasciitis, multiple organ failure, shock, and death. In the United States each year, from 50 to 100 previously healthy children or adults die from complications associated with their chickenpox illness.

Precautions against contamination

Vaccines are safe and effective. The FDA requires manufacturers to adhere to numerous procedures to protect its safety when producing vaccines. All vaccines undergo rigorous clinical trials for safety and effectiveness before being licensed by the FDA for use in the United States.

The FDA has many procedures in place, designed to detect and prevent the presence of adventitious agents in vaccines. These procedures include characterizations of the cell substrates used for vaccine production as well as testing the products by specified methods. For example, manufacturers today are required to test the cell lines (monkey kidney cells) used for the production of poliovirus vaccines for a variety of infectious agents: tuberculosis, SV40, herpes viruses (including simian cytomegalovirus), Coxsackie virus, lymphocytic choriomeningitis virus, measles, and others. Cell (tissue) culture tests must show an absence of cytopathogenic effects. Adult and suckling animals are also used to screen for viable microbial agents. A neurovirulence safety test is conducted for live oral poliovirus vaccine. The cell substrates used for measles/mumps/rubella (MMR) vaccine are derived from flocks free of avian leukosis virus. MMR vaccine also undergoes extensive testing for adventitious viral activity.

As technology improves, the FDA may require the application of new methods to screen for infectious agents in vaccines. Experimental assays have been applied by FDA on an ad hoc basis. For example, RT and PCR methods have been applied to some monopools (types) of polio vaccine to assure the absence of SIV and HIV. Other vaccines have been examined using other highly sensitive PCR methods.

7

Parents Should Be Allowed to Opt Out of Vaccinating Their Children

Barbara Loe Fisher

Barbara Loe Fisher is cofounder and president of the National Vaccine Information Center (NVIC), an organization formed in 1982 by parents whose children died or suffered injuries after being vaccinated. NVIC works to help parents whose children have suffered adverse reactions to vaccines, monitors vaccine research and public policy, and opposes compulsory vaccination laws.

Mandatory vaccination policies are most likely responsible for the recent increase in learning disabilities, mental retardation, autism, immune system disorders, and other long-term health problems. Children born into families with a history of autoimmune disorders or other genetic vulnerabilities are more likely to experience severe adverse reactions to vaccines—reactions that could eventually result in developmental disabilities and chronic illnesses. Yet medical researchers have largely ignored evidence linking vaccines to these health problems. The mainstream medical community prefers to assume that it is only coincidence when a vaccinated child comes down with a chronic disease, it insists that mandatory vaccination benefits society. This "one-size-fits-all" approach to immunization ignores the minority of children who are genetically vulnerable to vaccines and sacrifices their health for the public good. Parents should not be forced to submit to this inhumane public health policy.

Thank you for inviting me to share my thoughts about vaccine safety and communicate the concerns of thousands of mothers and fathers with vaccine injured children and those with well children, who contact the National Vaccine Information Center (NVIC) every year. I think it is also important to acknowledge that a number of prominent scientists and physicians from leading universities and hospitals in the US, Canada and

Europe spoke publicly about their vaccine safety concerns at the Second International Public Conference on Vaccination sponsored by our non-profit organization [in September 2000].

I am the mother of a now-grown son, my first-born, who was left with minimal brain damage following a convulsion, collapse-shock and state of unconsciousness within four hours of his fourth DPT [diphtheria/pertussis/tetanus] and OPV [oral polio vaccine] shots at age two and a half. The daughter of a nurse, the granddaughter of a doctor and a former writer at a teaching hospital before I became a mother [more than twenty] years ago, I thought I was an especially well educated woman when it came to science and medicine.

But, like most new mothers, I had no idea that vaccines carried any risk whatsoever. I'm not sure why I assumed vaccines were risk free, when I certainly knew that drugs and surgery entailed risks. Perhaps it had to do with the fact that vaccines are supposed to keep well people well. The concept of risk associated with a prevention is quite different from the concept of risk associated with a cure. At any rate, I believed vaccines were 100 percent safe and effective until my son, Chris, became a vaccine reaction statistic.

I am relating my experience because it is typical of the experiences you will hear from parents, who describe how their once healthy children became chronically ill following vaccination. Whether the vaccine reaction results in minimal brain damage, as was the case with my son, or more severe and profound brain damage, as is the case with those who have been awarded compensation under the National Childhood Vaccine Injury Act of 1986, there is a pattern and common experience that emerges. And that pattern and commonality of experience, reinforced over and over again with almost every vaccine reaction report, has contributed in no small way to why the vaccine safety issue will not go away, despite the concerted efforts by industry, government and medical organizations to convince the public that, when acute and chronic health problems follow vaccination, it is always just a coincidence.

Today's college educated, well read, internet-savvy health care consumer, who becomes a parent and whose child experiences a vaccine adverse event, has the opportunity that I did not have as a young mother in the 1980's to more quickly obtain information and then communicate with other parents who have shared the same experience. Like the biotechnology revolution, the mass communications revolution has created a national and international global network that shines a bright light on commonality of experience and gives immediacy and relevancy to it. That will continue to be true, even if government, industry and science continue to minimize the significance of that common experience.

An adverse reaction to the pertussis vaccine

In 1980, my son, Chris, was a healthy, cheerful, exceptionally bright two and a half year old child. A lively, contented baby who loved to be around people, he had begun saying words at seven months and speaking in full sentences at age two. At two and a half, he could identify the upper and lower case alphabet and numbers up to 20 and was beginning to identify words in the books we read together. He had memorized the deck of cards and created an interactive naming game he would play. One doctor told me he was cognitively gifted.

After his third DPT shot at seven months of age, there was a hard, red, hot lump that stayed at the site of the injection for several weeks. When I called my pediatrician's office, the nurse told me it was "a bad lot of DPT vaccine" but not to worry. My response was to ask "Should I bring him down for another one?" because I thought she meant the shot might not have been strong enough and I wanted my baby protected.

The day of his fourth DPT and OPV shots, Chris was healthy except for slight diarrhea that was left over from a 48 hour bout with the stomach flu he had at the beach three weeks earlier. The nurse giving him the shots said he didn't have a fever and that a little diarrhea didn't matter.

> *How many mothers are not in a child's presence to witness a serious vaccine reaction, which could easily occur in the middle of the night?*

When we got home, Chris seemed quieter than usual. Several hours later I walked into his bedroom to find him sitting in a rocking chair staring straight ahead as if he couldn't see me standing in the doorway. His face was white and his lips slightly blue, and when I called out his name, his eyes rolled back in his head, his head fell to his shoulder and it was like he had suddenly fallen asleep sitting up. I tried, but could not wake him. When I picked him up, he was like a dead weight and I carried him to his bed, where he stayed without moving for more than six hours, through dinnertime, until I called my Mom, who told me to immediately try to wake him, which I finally did with great difficulty. But he didn't know where he was, could not speak coherently and couldn't walk. I had to carry him to the bathroom and he fell asleep again in my arms and then slept for 12 more hours.

This was 1980. I had been given no information by my doctor about how to recognize a vaccine reaction. In the following days and weeks, Chris deteriorated physically, mentally and emotionally. He no longer knew his alphabet or numbers and would not look at the books we had once read together every day. He had no interest in his beloved deck of cards and had lost the ability to concentrate for more than a few seconds at a time. My once happy-go-lucky little boy was now listless and emotionally fragile, crying at the slightest frustration as if his heart would break.

Physically, the deterioration was just as profound. He had constant diarrhea that looked like attic foam insulation, became emaciated, stopped growing and was plagued with respiratory and ear infections for the first time in his life. Sometimes I would catch him staring and drooling slightly from one corner of his mouth. My Mom used the term "spaced out" to describe him. The pediatrician told me it was just a stage he was going through and not to worry about it. But after eight months of deterioration, I decided to take Chris to another pediatrician, who took one look at him and told me he might have either cystic fibrosis or celiac disease. All diagnostic tests came back negative. None of the doctors knew what was wrong with my son, who had become an entirely different child physically, mentally and emotionally.

It would be another year before I saw the television documentary "DPT: Vaccine Roulette," began research into the medical literature and found clinical descriptions of pertussis vaccine reactions in the pages of *Pediatrics,* the *New England Journal of Medicine, The Lancet,* and *British Medical Journal* which exactly matched the pertussis vaccine reaction symptoms I had seen my son suffer within four hours of his fourth DPT shot.

I learned that the British National Childhood Encephalopathy Study had found a statistically significant correlation between DPT vaccine and brain inflammation leading to chronic neurological damage and that the UCLA-FDA study had found that 1 in 875 DPT shots is followed within 48 hours by a convulsion or collapse/shock reaction just like my son had suffered.

I was stunned. I felt betrayed by a medical profession I had revered all my life.

The day my child reacted to the pertussis vaccine, he should have been in an emergency room, not unconscious in his bed. As his mother, I should have had the information I needed to recognize a vaccine reaction and take steps to deal with it, including calling my doctor and later making sure the reaction was recorded in his medical record and reported to the vaccine manufacturer and health officials.

Developmental disabilities and chronic health problems

At age six, when Chris could not learn to read or write, he was given an extensive battery of tests that confirmed minimal brain damage which took the form of multiple learning disabilities, including fine motor and short term memory delays; visual and auditory processing deficits; attention deficit disorder and other developmental problems. He was removed from the Montessori school he attended and placed in a self-contained classroom for the learning disabled in public school, where he stayed throughout elementary, junior and high school despite repeated efforts to mainstream him. Even with occupational therapy and counseling, he had a very negative educational experience, barely graduating from high school. As a young learning disabled adult, who blessedly survived the difficult teenage years without destroying himself like some of his learning disabled classmates, he is trying to find his place in the world, working in a mailroom and taking steps to better cope with the disabilities that made it difficult for him to learn in the classroom so he can get more formal education.

Has the increased administration of multiple vaccines . . . been an unrecognized co-factor in the epidemics of chronic disease and disability plaguing so many children today?

There is always the haunting vision of what would have been, intertwined with the certain knowledge that there is much to be thankful for. Both Chris and I know he was lucky compared to the children who have suffered vaccine reactions and been left quadriplegic, profoundly mentally retarded, epileptic or have died.

What I experienced as a young mother with my son is identical to the experiences of so many of the young mothers who today contact the National Vaccine Information Center. Mothers tell us how they took a happy, healthy, bright, normally developing child to the doctor to be vaccinated and then, within hours, days or weeks, their child regressed physically, mentally and emotionally and became a totally different child.

There may be a cumulative increased risk for vaccine-induced immune and brain dysfunction in genetically vulnerable children.

Many times, a mother will tell us that her baby exhibited acute symptoms within 72 hours of vaccination such as high pitched screaming or hours of constant crying sometimes alternating with extreme lethargy or long periods of unresponsiveness; head banging; twitching, jerking of the body or staring episodes; weakness or paralysis of one or more limbs; a dramatic change in eating and sleeping habits; loss of eye contact; restlessness; high fever; vomiting and diarrhea; body rash; or pronounced swelling, redness and heat at the site of the injection.

These acute symptoms are often followed by a gradual deterioration in overall health, a picture that includes chronic ear and respiratory infections and onset of multiple allergies, including asthma; loss of appetite and persistent diarrhea; sleep disturbances that turn night into day and day into night; loss of developmental milestones like the ability to roll over or sit up; older children will complain of muscle weakness, joint pain and disabling fatigue and exhibit loss of memory and loss of previously demonstrated cognitive abilities, speech or physical skills; development of strange or violent behavior that includes hyperactivity, screaming, biting, hitting, social withdrawal, and obsessively repetitive movements such as flapping, rubbing, rocking and spinning.

The once healthy, normally developing child becomes a totally different, sick child. And the mother, who carried that child inside her for nine months and nursed that baby after birth and whose every waking moment is connected to preserving the well-being of that child, knows her child in a way no one else does. The mother knows with all of her senses that her child changed and is different now, even if she doesn't know why. It is a powerful experience, grounded in a primal love and instinct to nurture and protect her young.

A problematic vaccine policy

Depending on the child and therapy interventions available, there is either gradual full recovery or the child is eventually diagnosed with varying degrees of permanent brain and immune system dysfunction ranging from severe and profound mental retardation and medication resistant seizure disorders, autistic behaviors, learning disabilities, attention deficit hyperactivity disorder or other chronic health problems. Upon questioning, many parents reveal that their child suffered previous vaccine reaction symptoms that were dismissed by their doctor as unrelated or unimportant. Others report their child was sick at the time of vaccination. Others report a strong family history of autoimmune disease. Still other babies, especially those whose vaccine reactions are followed by death, were born premature, were underweight or had a history of health problems prior to repeated vaccination.

In other words, these are children who have potentially identifiable genetic or other biological high risk factors which are not being factored into a one-size-fits-all national vaccine policy that today allows a baby to be injected with 9 or more vaccines on one day. The relatively small new vaccine pre-licensure studies do not include these categories of children routinely vaccinated in America, including premature, underweight and sick babies and those who have suffered previous vaccine reactions.

But how many children who react and become chronically ill are we talking about? Is it really only 1 in a 110,000 or 1 in a million who are left permanently disabled after vaccine reactions? Former FDA Commissioner David Kessler observed in 1993 that less than one percent of doctors report adverse events following prescription drug use. There have been estimates that perhaps less than 10 percent of doctors report hospitalizations, injuries, deaths or other serious health problems following vaccination. There are about 12,000 reports made to the Vaccine Adverse Event Reporting System every year. If the number 12,000 only represents 10 percent of what is occurring, then the real number may be 120,000 vaccine adverse events. If 12,000 reports represents only one percent of the actual total, then the real number may be 1.2 million vaccine adverse events annually. Yes, it is illogical to assume that all reported adverse events following vaccination *are* causally related. But is it not just as illogical to assume that most events are *not?*

It would be medically useful as well as more humane to find out why some children . . . respond adversely to vaccination.

If I had not walked into my child's room when I did, I would not have witnessed the post-pertussis vaccine convulsion, collapse shock and six hour state of unconsciousness which, not counting the few minutes I was able to rouse my son to a state of semi-consciousness, was actually an 18 hour state of altered consciousness. If Chris had been a four month old baby and not a precocious two and a half year old, the regression he underwent following vaccination may not have been so immediately and dramatically apparent. How many mothers are not in a child's presence to witness a serious vaccine reaction, which could easily occur in the middle of the night? And how many infants are regressing after vaccine reactions but are never diagnosed until long after the damage has occurred, thereby preventing even a temporal relationship between vaccination and neuro-immune dysfunction from being recognized?

Today, as vaccination rates with DTP, polio, MMR [measles/mumps/rubella] and Hib [haemophilus influenzae type b] vaccines approach 98 percent for children entering kindergarten, those once common child-hood infectious diseases have disappeared. My mother had whooping cough as a child and, as a nurse, took care of children on polio wards. I had rubella, measles and chicken pox and, in 1955, lined up in grade school to get my first dose of Salk polio vaccine. Mass vaccination with measles vaccine has driven the numbers of cases of measles down from more than 400,000 cases in 1965 to less than 100 in 1999. And the dreaded polio has been eradicated from our nation.

But individual and public health is not measured solely by an absence of infectious disease. Today, instead of epidemics of measles and polio, our children are experiencing epidemics of chronic disease and disability. In the past 20 years, rates of asthma and attention deficit disorder have more than doubled; diabetes and learning disabilities have tripled; and autism has increased by 300 percent or more in most states. Our public school systems are unable to build or staff special education classrooms fast enough to serve the millions of chronically disabled and ill children and the 425 billion dollar annual health care price tag to treat chronic disease continues to climb.

An unrecognized cause of chronic disease

The larger unanswered question is: has the increased administration of multiple vaccines in the first three years of life, when the brain and im-mune systems develop most rapidly, been an unrecognized co-factor in the epidemics of chronic disease and disability plaguing so many children today?

Other potential co-factors are increased exposures to pesticides, chemicals and other environmental toxins; overuse of antibiotics and other pharmaceuticals; nutritionally compromised food sources and un-healthy lifestyles. But there is a compelling argument to be made that the dramatic increase in chronic brain and immune dysfunction in children, especially the rising number of reports of regression in previously healthy children, is due to an early exposure that is being experienced by all chil-dren but which is harming an expanding minority of them.

Genetic factors alone have been suggested as a cause for autism in-creases, for example. But if the presence of certain genes were the sole causal factor for autism, in order to explain the huge increase in autism in the past two decades, there would have had to be a significant genetic shift in the whole population. A more likely explanation is that the pres-ence of certain genes, together with one or more new environmental ex-posures which act as triggers, account for the increases in autism and other chronic diseases in childhood.

Many biological responses are at least partially under genetic control. If, for example, adverse responses to vaccination are tied to the genes re-sponsible for predisposition to autoimmunity and immune-mediated neurological dysfunction, then it is possible that the addition of more doses of vaccines to the routine schedule in the past two decades has af-fected more and more children with that genetic predisposition. With each dose of vaccine or simultaneous injection of multiple vaccines, there may be a cumulative increased risk for vaccine-induced immune and brain dysfunction in genetically vulnerable children. So the pool of genetically susceptible children has not changed but the environmental triggers have increased. Therefore, when all children only were exposed to DPT and polio vaccine in the 1960's, a tiny fraction of the genetically susceptibles responded adversely. But with the addition of measles, mumps, and rubella to the routine schedule in 1979, and then Hib, hepatitis B and chicken pox in the late 1980's and 1990's, far more of the genetically susceptibles have been brought into the vaccine adverse responder group.

My son, born in 1978, was part of the first bubble that turned into a tidal wave of learning disabled, hyperactive, autistic children that required the creation of special classrooms in the public school system to deal with this new phenomenon. Were he and his classmates the canaries in the coal mine, ignored because, as German immunologist Wolfgang Ehrengut once suggested "What must not be, cannot be?" Certainly, the *a priori* assumption that increased use of multiple doses of vaccines over the past quarter century has played no role in the rise in chronic disease and disability in children is as unscientific and potentially dangerous as the assumption that an individual child's regression following vaccination is only coincidentally and not causally related to vaccination, especially in the absence of basic science research into the biological mechanisms of vaccine-induced injury. Without pathological profiles to conclusively determine what is and is not a vaccine-induced event, the coincidence assumption will continue to be used to maintain the status quo, with all the inherent risks that assumption carries with it.

Epidemiological studies will be fatally flawed by the coincidence assumption in the absence of objective, science-based criteria for determining what is and is not vaccine-induced. This is especially true when, for the past 35 years, virtually all American children have been vaccinated with at least DPT and polio vaccines. Therefore, the true background rates in vaccinated children for mental retardation, medication resistant seizure disorders, learning disabilities, attention deficit hyperactivity disorder, asthma, diabetes and other chronic disease, is unknown.

Forced vaccination . . . is a de facto selection and sacrifice of the genetically vulnerable in the name of the public good.

The two previous Institute of Medicine committees charged by Congress with evaluating the medical literature for evidence that vaccines can cause injury and death pointed out "There are many gaps and limitations in knowledge bearing directly or indirectly on the safety of vaccines." Little has changed in the landscape of vaccine reaction research since that assessment was made. And yet, the medical literature dating back to the turn of the twentieth century is already rich with evidence documenting that the complications of vaccines containing lab altered viruses and bacteria are often identical to the complications of the infectious diseases caused by those same viruses and bacteria. From smallpox and polio to pertussis and rubella, the brain and immune system changes due to complications of disease is quite similar to that following complications of vaccination.

When you look at the possible biological mechanisms for vaccine-induced neuro-immune dysfunction, in addition to genetic factors, the picture is complicated by the presence of heavy metals in vaccines, such as the preservative mercury and the adjuvant aluminum. And there are other vaccine components, such as MSG and formalin that, together with residual DNA and possible adventitious agent contamination from animal human cell substrates, have unknown biological effects. In addition, atypical introduction of viruses and bacteria through vaccination has yet to be evaluated for the long term effect on chromosomal integrity and this is worth looking at as the past two generations of highly vaccinated children give birth to their children.

The need for humane vaccine policies

But what do we do if increased vaccination in childhood is contributing to increased chronic disease and disability in childhood? Some would view this as an unacceptable catastrophe for vaccination programs and public perception of them. This fear may be one reason why there hasn't been a funding commitment to conduct basic science and applied vaccine adverse event research. If you don't really look, you don't have to deal with what you find.

But, in the long run, we have far less to fear by honestly searching for the truth and dealing with it now, than we do by failing to see the canaries dying in the mine before we take steps to modify vaccine policies to make them safer and more humane. It would be medically useful as well as more humane to find out why some children, like my son, respond adversely to vaccination. It would be useful to understand what common genetic and other host factors are shared by vaccine adverse responders, both those who fail to mount an antibody response and those who react, so that identification and screening techniques could be developed to spare their lives. With the human genome project yielding invaluable information, the more precise identification of individuals at increased genetic or other biological risk for responding adversely to vaccination would go a long way toward reassuring the individual mother that everything possible has been done to minimize the vaccine risk for her child.

The anecdotal evidence we have gathered for two decades suggests that a significant portion of vaccine injury and death may be prevented if children who exhibit acute severe reactions, especially those who suffer chronic health problems following vaccination, were not re-vaccinated; and if more caution were exercised when vaccinating premature and sick babies and children with personal or strong family histories of autoimmune or neurological disease, especially with regard to giving them multiple vaccines on one day.

This, of course, would require vaccine policies to abandon a one-size-fits-all approach, which has proven to be ill advised in many other areas of medicine. It would require re-thinking the mission of achieving a 100 percent vaccination rate with every vaccine and an institutional commitment to rejecting the idea that some children are expendable in order to achieve the mission.

The utilitarian pseudo-ethic, a politically motivated philosophical ra-

tionale used by the US Supreme Court to justify the state-ordered steriliza-
tion of a mentally retarded girl in 1927, but finally discredited as inher-
ently immoral at Nuremberg in 1947, is being used today by public health
officials to persuade states to force vaccination with informed consent.
The argument is that all must take the risk for the greater good. However,
the as yet unidentified genetic factors involved in vaccine injury and
death means that vaccine risks are not being equally shared by all. Therefore, forced vaccination and the achievement of a 100 percent vaccination
rate is a de facto selection and sacrifice of the genetically vulnerable in the
name of the public good. And when it is your child and your family being
dismissed as expendable, the full horror of why utilitarianism should
never be used to justify public policy becomes very clear.

This brings me to the recent article published in the *Journal of the American Medical Association*, asserting that religious and philosophical exemptions to vaccination are endangering the public health and should be eliminated or severely restricted. Doctors, say CDC officials, should be given the
power to sit in judgment on the depth and sincerity of a parent's spiritual
and conscientiously held beliefs. It is a chilling specter and one that is
adding to distrust and fear of public health officials who have decided, with
this arrogant stance, to further polarize an already polarized issue.

My second son, who is graduating with high honors from high
school and heading for college [in 2002], was vaccinated at age four with
DT and polio vaccines and developed a pseudo tumor of the brain, from
which he thankfully recovered with little residual damage. In my family,
we do not have a history of neurological disease, convulsions or learning
disabilities but we do have a history of serious autoimmune disorders, including rheumatoid arthritis, lupus, thyroid disease, diabetes and life
threatening allergies to prescription drugs. There is no doubt in my mind
that my children are genetically predisposed to adverse responses to vaccination but the CDC and AAP vaccine policies do not allow for medical
exemptions for my children.

The result of policy without compassion

I am not alone. There are mothers, whose children have suffered vaccine
reactions, who are being coerced by doctors to continue vaccinating with
the threat that they will be reported to social services as child abusers and
their children taken from them if they don't comply. Children have been
denied an education and denied health insurance by HMO's and government entitlement benefits by agencies persuaded to employ a no vaccination, no health insurance and benefit policy. The mothers of these children know they have a sacred duty to protect their children's lives and
they live in fear of state officials and even their own pediatricians. The
only legal protection they have is to exercise a religious or conscientious
belief exemption to vaccination.

How can a humane and just society force a mother against her will to
violate her spiritual and conscientiously held beliefs and risk her child's
life in the name of the public good? What state official or doctor can
claim that moral imperative under any circumstance?

And if the informed consent ethic, which has been the gold standard
in the ethical practice of medical care since World War II, is totally aban-

doned and replaced with state-forced risk taking that results in the sacrifice of the genetically vulnerable, what precedent does that set for all public policy which can be justified by government officials in the name of the greater good?

The more health officials and doctors force, rather than persuade, people to do what they want them to do, the more fearful and hostile the people will become. The more the reality of vaccine reactions, injuries and deaths is denied and minimized, the more distrustful the people will become. At a 1984 meeting of the Redbook Committee of the American Academy of Pediatrics, where we were discussing the framework for the table of compensable events that would become a centerpiece of the 1986 National Childhood Vaccine Injury Act, I said: "A system that will not bend, will break."

Seventeen years later, there is growing evidence that ideology not tempered with restraint and grounded in good science; inflexible administration of policy without compassion; refusal to allow informed, voluntary risk taking; dismissal of the suffering of individuals who are casualties of the program, all combine to destroy public confidence in and support of the mass vaccination system no matter how many advertising dollars are spent to promote the benefits and minimize the risks of vaccination.

You have a formidable task ahead of you and there are no easy answers. On your shoulders rests the hopes of mothers and fathers with children who have been hurt by vaccines and those who want their healthy children to stay healthy. What you choose to do, the guidance you choose to give at this crossroads, before scores of new vaccines are brought to market and mandated in the next decade, may well determine if the mass vaccination system in this country will bend or break.

My prayers and the prayers of every mother and father I know are with you.

8

Parents Should Not Be Allowed to Opt Out of Vaccinating Their Children

Steven P. Shelov

Steven P. Shelov, a practicing pediatrician, is chair of the Department of Pediatrics, Babies' and Children's Hospital at the Maimonides Medical Center in New York City.

Children's immunization programs should not be optional. Failure to vaccinate a child would greatly increase his or her risk of contracting dangerous infectious diseases; it would also expose other children to illness and possibly lead to a deadly epidemic. On occasion children do have mild negative reactions to vaccines, but severe adverse reactions are extremely rare. Furthermore, there is no evidence linking vaccines to disorders such as autism, sudden infant death syndrome, multiple sclerosis, or asthma. The hazards associated with illnesses such as tetanus, measles, and polio are far greater than the risks posed by immunization. Allowing parents to opt out of vaccinating their children would endanger public health.

Some parents today are in a quandary regarding the need for immunizing their children. They need not be.

True, recent media stories about an increase in childhood autism associated with immunizations and other illnesses have led some to question the need to give their children the full range of vaccinations required by most school districts in the country. In addition, numerous others have had unfortunate experiences with their own children or relatives with respect to a bad reaction to an immunization. Yet, it is important to keep all these issues and incidents in perspective and not to erode public confidence in immunizing our children. In fact, if the U.S. population or any population regards immunizing children as optional, we risk having large numbers of children becoming vulnerable to the most deadly diseases known to man. As a practicing pediatrician, I am passionately opposed to that. The following are a few questions some skeptical parents are asking about the vaccination issue:

What would happen if I did not have my child immunized? Without immunizations there would be a significant possibility that your child would contract some of the diseases that are now waiting to come back. These include: whooping cough (pertussis), tetanus, polio, measles, mumps, German measles (rubella), bacterial meningitis and diphtheria.

These illnesses all may injure children severely, leaving them deaf, blind, paralyzed or they even may cause death. For example, in 1960 there were more than 1.5 million cases of measles and more than 400 deaths associated with this disease. As a result of our active immunization process in 1998 the United States had only 89 cases of measles and there were no deaths.

If the U.S. population . . . regards immunizing children as optional, we risk having large numbers of children becoming vulnerable to the most deadly diseases known to man.

Why should I accept any risk of immunization for my child when other children already are immunized? Won't that protect my child? It is important to understand the concept of herd immunity and public health vs. individual risk. Individual risk is always a possibility with any procedure, medication, new activity or vaccine. The key to any program or new intervention is to minimize the risk. There is no question that vaccines are the safest, most risk-free type of medication ever developed. Nevertheless, occasionally—very occasionally—children have been known to experience a bad, or adverse, reaction to a vaccine. In some cases—polio vaccine, for example—one in 1 million doses appears to have been associated with vaccine-related mild polio disease. The reactions to other vaccines also have been very, very small, though nevertheless significant for the child or family who have experienced one.

It is not, however, good public policy to give those few at-risk situations priority over the goal of protecting the population as a whole from those diseases. If the pool of unimmunized children becomes large enough, then the disease itself may reemerge in those unimmunized children, possibly in epidemic proportions. This has occurred in countries where immunizations have been allowed to decrease; most recently pertussis (whooping cough) resurfaced in Europe. Failure to immunize a child not only puts that child at risk of illness but also increases the potential for harm to other children who are not able to be vaccinated because they are too young or too ill or to those who in rare cases are vaccinated but the vaccination fails to provide the expected protection.

Protecting children's health

Are immunizations safe? Don't they hurt? Reactions to vaccines may occur, but they usually are mild. Serious reactions are very, very rare but also may occur. Remember, the risks from these potentially dangerous childhood illnesses are far greater than any risk of serious reaction from immunization. Even though immunizations may hurt a little when they are given, and your baby may cry for a few minutes, and there might be some swelling, protecting your child's health is worth a few tears and a little temporary discomfort.

Isn't it better that children get a disease such as chicken pox to give them a permanent immunity? If a child gets the disease, the danger is that the child may develop serious complications from the disease. The immunity conferred following the recommended immunization schedule will give excellent immunity and not place the child at risk.

Is it true that hepatitis B vaccine can cause autism or juvenile diabetes, sudden infant death syndrome, or SIDS, multiple sclerosis or asthma? There have been occasional reports in the media associating this vaccine with all of the above illnesses. Scientific research has not found any evidence linking the hepatitis B vaccine to autism, SIDS, multiple sclerosis, juvenile diabetes or asthma. In fact, SIDS rates have declined during the same time period that the hepatitis B vaccine has been recommended for routine immunization. Although some media have circulated reports that health authorities in France have stopped giving the hepatitis vaccine to children, that is not true. French health officials did not stop giving the hepatitis vaccine but decided not to administer the vaccine in the schools and recommended that the vaccine be given in medical settings.

Is there a link between measles vaccine and autism? No. There is no scientifically proven link between measles vaccine and autism. Autism is a chronic developmental disorder often first identified in toddlers ages 18 months to 30 months. The MMR (mumps, measles, rubella vaccine) is administered just before the peakage of autism that has caused some parents to assume a causal relationship, but a recent study in a British journal showed there was no association between the MMR vaccine and autism.

Vaccines are the safest, most risk-free type of medication ever developed.

It is assumed that there has been an increase in the diagnosis of autism because the definition for who would fall under that category has changed. In addition, parents and medical professionals are more aware of this condition and are more likely to pursue that diagnosis. Though there may be an increase in the number of children who have autism, there have been many studies completed that show that the MMR does not cause autism.

Aren't measles, mumps and rubella relatively harmless illnesses? Measles is a highly contagious respiratory disease. It causes a rash, high fever, cough and runny nose. In addition, it can cause encephalitis, which leads to convulsions, deafness or mental retardation in one to two children of every 2,000 who get it. Of every 1,000 people who get measles, one to two will die. MMR can prevent this disease. Mumps is less serious than measles but may cause fever, headache and swelling of one or both sides of the jaw. Four to 6 percent of those who get mumps will get meningitis, which puts the child at risk for significant disability and potential retardation. In addition, inflammation of the testicles occurs in four of every 10 adult males who get mumps, and mumps may result in hearing loss that usually is permanent. The effects of rubella are mild in children and adults—causing only a minor rash—but the major reason to prevent rubella in the community is to prevent exposure of pregnant women to children who have rubella. When contracted by a pregnant woman, rubella may infect her unborn baby, leading to a significant potential for mental retardation and a host of serious defects. This devastating disease, known as congenital rubella syndrome, essentially has been eliminated with the use of rubella vaccine.

The need for continued vaccination

Given that measles, rubella and mumps essentially have disappeared from the United States and therefore are uncommon, why should we continue to immunize? The measles virus continues to be present in other countries outside the United States. Given the large number of immigrants to this country, the potential for exposure to measles remains a real potential. Just a few weeks ago [in early 2000] several young children who recently emigrated from the United Kingdom came into one of our pediatrician's offices. Due to the decrease in immunization vigilance in the United Kingdom against measles, these young children were infected with measles, and they put at risk the other infants and children in the waiting room of this busy pediatrician's office. If those other children contract measles, they will be at risk for developing serious sequela of the disease. And, should they develop the disease, they potentially will expose others as well. A mini-epidemic could have been caused by these infected children with measles.

Should parents be able to choose not to vaccinate their child without being barred from enrolling that child in school? Immunizing children is a public-health issue. Public-health laws in all 50 states require immunization of children as a condition of school enrollment. This is as it should be, since public health must take precedence. Immunizations have a clear community benefit and, therefore, individual preferences should not be permitted to expose the public to the hazards of infectious diseases.

In summary, it is clear that the risk of exposing children to infectious disease should there be a decline in immunizations is a risk to which the population of the United States should not be exposed. It always is regrettable when an individual case of an adverse event occurs no matter what might have taken place. These adverse events clearly affect the child and obviously the family as well, and there indeed is always an outcry when this does occur. However, as with all safe, proven interventions, an exception could always occur given a normal risk ratio.

It would be actual malpractice and poor public-health philosophy and practice to consider not immunizing our children against the potentially deadly infectious diseases. We should be thankful to our research scientists, epidemiologists, and medical and pharmaceutical industry for the skill and care with which these important vaccines have been developed and the care with which the vaccine policies have been developed and monitored. There is no question in my mind that immunizations are one of the most important ways parents can protect their children against serious diseases. Without immunizations the children of the United States would be exposed to deadly diseases that continue to occur throughout the world.

9

The Smallpox Vaccine Should Be Administered on a Voluntary Basis

Jonathan Rauch

Jonathan Rauch is a senior writer for National Journal *and the author of* Government's End: Why Washington Stopped Working.

One of the most serious bioterrorist threats today is smallpox. Since routine smallpox immunization ended in the 1970s, supplies of smallpox vaccine have dwindled, and the vast majority of the U.S. population is currently susceptible to the disease. The government is working to increase its smallpox-vaccine inventory, yet experts continue to debate whether routine vaccinations should resume. If all Americans were required to be immunized, thousands would die or suffer serious side effects from the vaccine. Some analysts have suggested an alternative "containment strategy" which would focus on quarantining and vaccinating people in the immediate vicinity of a smallpox outbreak. But this strategy is risky—any missteps could enable the virus to spread. Rather than compulsory immunization or containment, individuals themselves should be allowed to decide if they should be vaccinated against smallpox.

On the days following the terrorist attacks that brought down the World Trade Center and demolished part of the Pentagon, I received a series of e-mails from my sister asking what I thought she could do to protect herself and her family. Should she stock up on water? On food? What about buying a gas mask? I told her I doubted that any of those things would really help. At first blush the notion of suburban moms buying gas masks seemed a little silly. But a lot of people were buying gas masks at that point, and mostly they were not silly people, and the impulse they were acting on was not silly. What they wanted was to do something: to exert at least a little control over a new and frightening situation. That is just the sort of impulse that the fight against terrorism needs to put to use. One way to use it is against the threat of smallpox.

Experts have agreed that smallpox terrorism is potentially the Big One. Maybe not bigger in terms of lives lost than, say, a nuclear warhead detonating over Manhattan, but certainly right up there, and probably more socially destabilizing. Unlike chemical agents and some other biological agents, such as anthrax (as we've lately seen) and botulism, smallpox spreads virulently from person to person. The disease is fatal 30 percent of the time and leaves its survivors disfigured and sometimes blind. Symptoms take a week or two to appear. In an urbanized country full of planes, trains, and automobiles, smallpox could easily spread to any number of cities and states before health officials realized what was going on.

Routine smallpox vaccination ended in the early 1970s, because a worldwide campaign had succeeded in eradicating the disease. The virus survived only in laboratories in the United States and the Soviet Union. After the Soviet Union collapsed, credible reports surfaced alleging that the Soviets had produced smallpox in large quantities, for biological warfare. Bio-terrorism experts began to worry that the Russians might have let the virus slip into the wrong hands. Still, most people believed that smallpox's very virulence made it an unlikely weapon of terror. After September 11, 2001, a lot of those people changed their minds.

The problem with the smallpox vaccine

I was vaccinated for smallpox years ago, in childhood; so were many other Americans who are now over thirty. But it's unclear how much good this would do if smallpox were unleashed today. "One of the problems with smallpox vaccine is that immunity doesn't last very long," Peter J. Hotez, a senior fellow at the Sabin Vaccine Institute, in Washington, D.C., told me when I asked if I would be safe. "It can last as few as three to five years." And younger people, of course, weren't vaccinated. America today would be a tinderbox for smallpox: something like 90 percent of the population is thought to be susceptible.

America today would be a tinderbox for smallpox: something like 90 percent of the population is thought to be susceptible.

To its credit, the Clinton Administration took the threat seriously. Realizing that existing stocks (about 12 million to 15 million doses of twenty-year-old vaccine) were too thin to cope with a serious crisis, in September of 2000 the government ordered up a new smallpox vaccine, with the first 40 million doses to be delivered in 2004 and more to come thereafter. In October 2001, as anthrax scares transformed the threat of bio-terrorism into reality, the Bush Administration announced that it would seek to increase the smallpox-vaccine inventory to 300 million doses, possibly by 2002.

With the new vaccine will come a new and difficult question: Who should be vaccinated? My first thought was "Everyone." Or at least—as Homeland Security Chief Tom Ridge has suggested—we should resume routine vaccination of children. But this sort of uniform approach has a significant drawback. The smallpox vaccine is not perfectly safe. During the eradication campaign, according to Tara O'Toole, of the Johns Hopkins School of Public Health, about one in 300,000 people died from side effects of the vaccine or suffered irreversible brain damage. At that rate, if all 280 million Americans were to be vaccinated, nearly a thousand people would die or be gravely injured.

[Let] individual people and doctors, rather than public-health authorities, decide who would be vaccinated.

For that reason the government instead built its plans around a containment strategy. Vaccine would be stockpiled for use in case of an outbreak. If smallpox were spotted, authorities would declare a health emergency and rush to vaccinate (or quarantine) everyone likely to have crossed the virus's path. (Fortunately, the vaccine is effective even when given a few days after exposure, so in principle post-outbreak vaccination could stop the spread.) There is certainly something to be said for the containment strategy, but it is not without worrisome risks. It relies on health workers, public officials, and the public itself to react quickly, calmly, and efficiently. Virtually everyone who was exposed would need to be promptly vaccinated or quarantined. That would be easier said than done, because the early symptoms of smallpox look like flu. Moreover, once word of a smallpox outbreak hit the street, panic, chaos, flight, and human error would inevitably give the virus chances to spread. Even if a containment plan ran like clockwork, some people—those caught at the onset—would die who might have lived had they previously been vaccinated.

Voluntary vaccination

While I was pondering these problems, I came across a news article from October of 2000, in which a biologist named Paul W. Ewald, of Amherst College, suggested something so obvious that no one else seemed to have considered it. He proposed making the smallpox vaccine available to the public, the way many other vaccines are today. Individuals could then decide, after being apprised of the risks and with medical advice, whether or not to get themselves and their children inoculated.

Regular readers of the *Atlantic Monthly* may recall from an article in the February, 1999, issue—"A New Germ Theory," by Judith Hooper—that Ewald has specialized in thinking about how doctors can use evolutionary pressures to make pathogens more benign, and how terrorists might contrive to make pathogens deadlier. That led him to think about smallpox. I called Ewald recently and asked him to expand on the idea of voluntary vaccination.

"I think the key thing that's been missed in this analysis," he told me, "is that the more any given vaccine is used, the less bang the terrorist is going to get." Even if only a minority of the public chose vaccination, those people's immunity would not only protect them in the event of an attack but would also slow transmission to others. That could buy precious time. Moreover, if, say, 30 million people were vaccinated, there would be 30 million fewer to vaccinate in a crisis. Indeed, Ewald said, "If you have thirty million people vaccinated, the terrorists might just decide, Let's not bother." The terrorists might, of course, try something else—but pretty much anything would be better than smallpox.

"Another problem," Ewald said, "is that if you wait until the crisis is at hand, you lose a chance to have careful analysis on a patient-by-patient basis of the risks posed by vaccinating. It might just be that you're cranking out vaccinations as fast as possible." There is a deeper point here as well. People are as different in their tolerance for risk as they are in their tolerance for vaccines. To weigh the minuscule but real risk of a smallpox attack against the minuscule but real risk of complications from a vaccine is to weigh imponderables. No public-health expert is any more qualified to make this call than is the person who will have to live with the consequences.

It isn't surprising that it was a biologist who suggested letting individual people and doctors, rather than public-health authorities, decide who would be vaccinated. Biologists tend to see a world of variegated individuals, whereas the public-health establishment tends to view the public as a "population" and to think in terms of centralized, one-size-fits-all measures based on expert knowledge. A national anti-terror campaign will certainly need its share of unitary, top-down strategies on the public-health and national-defense models; but if it is to be sustainable and successful it will need to treat the public first and foremost as a resource to be enlisted, not merely as a population to be instructed. As we know from United Airlines Flight 93, engaging the intelligence and moral judgment of ordinary people can make all the difference.[1] Why not apply that lesson to the greatest terrorist threat of all?

1. Flight 93 was one of the planes hijacked by terrorists on September 11, 2001. It is believed that the terrorists had intended to crash the plane into the White House. Their plans were thwarted by the counteractions of passengers, and the plane crashed into a field in rural Pennsylvania.

10

The Smallpox Vaccine Should Not Be Administered on a Voluntary Basis

Henry I. Miller

Henry I. Miller is a fellow at the Hoover Institution and the author of To America's Health: A Proposal to Reform the Food and Drug Administration.

In the wake of the September 11, 2001, terrorist attack on the United States, polls indicate that 60 percent of Americans would choose to be immunized against smallpox if the vaccine were widely available. But voluntary immunization would be unwise, because the smallpox vaccine can cause serious adverse effects, including disfiguring rashes, encephalitis, neurological damage, and death. A more effective strategy for containing an outbreak of smallpox would be to quarantine all infected individuals and vaccinate everyone who may have come in contact with the disease. Public health authorities can be trusted to respond appropriately to bioterrorist attacks involving smallpox.

S ixty percent of Americans would opt for smallpox immunization if the vaccine were available, according to a recent poll, and U.S. health officials have just negotiated the purchase of enough vaccine for everyone in the United States. Those two facts may be a prescription for bad medicine.

Medically and epidemiologically, smallpox is the most feared and potentially devastating of all infectious agents. It spreads from person to person, primarily via droplets coughed up by infected persons, via direct contact, and from contaminated clothing and bed linens. Smallpox is fatal in approximately a third of previously unvaccinated persons who contract the disease.

During the last weeks of 2001, the media have raised the specter of terrorists using smallpox virus as a weapon. The German government has bought six million doses of vaccine, and pressure is mounting in the United States for widespread, or even universal, vaccination. (Routine smallpox

From "A Smallpox Shot in the Dark," by Henry I. Miller, *The Scientist*, January 21, 2002. Copyright © 2002 by *The Scientist*. Reprinted with permission.

vaccinations ceased in this country in 1972.) The U.S. government has ordered 300 million doses of the vaccine, and at a recent hearing, U.S. Sen. Arlen Specter (R-Pa.) said it is just "common sense" to make it available to everyone who wants it.

Is voluntary vaccination appropriate?

But is it really? The live vaccine consists of live vaccinia virus, which is closely related to smallpox virus. Impure and crude by the modern standards of recombinant DNA-derived, or gene-spliced, vaccines such as those that have been successfully deployed against hepatitis B since the 1980s, the smallpox vaccine is not very different from the one introduced by the English physician Edward Jenner in the 18th century. It can provoke various serious side effects, including rashes; spreading from the inoculation site to face, eyelid, mouth or genitalia, and generalized infection. Approximately one in every 300,000 vaccinations causes encephalitis, which can lead to permanent neurological damage; and between one and three in every million die. Thus, vaccinating the entire population would be expected to kill as many as a thousand Americans, and maim and disfigure many others. Moreover, that assumes that the newer, ostensibly incrementally improved versions of the vaccinia vaccine are no less safe: Federal regulators have been uncharacteristically lax about requiring evidence of safety and efficacy in a drug intended for healthy individuals.

Control [of smallpox] depends on early detection, quarantine of infected individuals, surveillance of contacts, and focused, aggressive vaccination of all possible contacts.

If the re-emergence of smallpox were likely, vaccination would be appropriate. However, smallpox virus no longer occurs in nature but is limited to two known, legitimate repositories, one in the United States, the other in Russia (and perhaps to illegitimate ones in several other countries). It is, therefore, very difficult to obtain, and also to cultivate and disseminate.

Also, smallpox is not immediately contagious after infection. It can be transmitted from one person to another only after a one- to two-week incubation period and the appearance of the characteristic rash, by which time the victim is prostrate, bedridden, and probably hospitalized. Therefore, the much-publicized scenario in which suicide terrorists infect themselves and then spread the disease widely through the population is not a realistic one. And although universal smallpox vaccination was phased out throughout the world during the 1970s, individuals who were vaccinated prior to that time retain significant immunity from these immunizations, both against contracting the disease and against a fatal outcome in case of infection. Scientists know a great deal about the long-term retention of immunity from a landmark study of 1,163 smallpox cases in Liverpool in 1902–1903. Among those infected, 7% of the people

50 or older who had received the vaccine as children experienced severe disease and death, while 26% of unvaccinated people in that age group contracted serious cases of smallpox and all died.

Even if an outbreak were to occur, public health authorities know how to respond. Control depends on early detection, quarantine of infected individuals, surveillance of contacts, and focused, aggressive vaccination of all possible contacts—an approach dubbed "quarantine-ring vaccination." Approximately 15 million doses of smallpox vaccine are available in the United States, and data suggest that these would still be effective if diluted fivefold, to yield 75 million.

Moreover, the federal government has taken steps to cope with the possibility of a terrorist attack involving smallpox by educating doctors to recognize the disease and by vaccinating small teams of experts who can rush to any part of the country to confirm the diagnosis and contain and treat an outbreak. The city of New York has begun to map out various locations where residents would go to be immunized should mass vaccinations be necessary.

In summary, given the difficulty of estimating the risks and benefits of vaccinating against a nonexistent disease using a vaccine that carries known, serious, sometimes-lethal side effects, one must agree with the conclusion of David Busch, head of infectious diseases at California Pacific Medical Center in San Francisco. "It's inappropriate" to vaccinate the entire country for a disease whose threat is only theoretical, and immunization should only be given "as needed, not as desired."

If federal officials act otherwise, they will be more in the realm of public relations than public health. Even the expenditure of upwards of a billion dollars to stockpile 300 million doses of smallpox vaccine is arguably in the category of political cover. Far better, surely, to use those resources to ensure that susceptible Americans are immunized against common and life-threatening infectious diseases such as influenza, hepatitis, and pneumococcal pneumonia. (Flu alone kills 20,000 in an average year.)

Sherlock Holmes admonished in *A Scandal in Bohemia* that "it is a capital mistake to theorize before one has data." It is worse to make the wrong decision after one has data.

11

An Improved Anthrax Vaccine Is Needed

Brian Vastag

Science journalist Brian Vastag is a senior media relations representative for the Office of Communications and Public Affairs at Johns Hopkins Medical Institutions.

The anthrax mail attacks of the fall of 2001 prompted many requests for anthrax vaccinations. While the currently available vaccine is effective, it does have drawbacks, such as painful multiple injections and some adverse effects. For example, some analysts maintain that the anthrax vaccine could cause chronic fatigue, memory loss, and other severe reactions. An investigative arm of the Institute of Medicine (IOM) concluded that the anthrax vaccine is not linked with any chronic ailments, yet it is possible that serious adverse reactions have been underreported. Immunologists need to develop an improved anthrax vaccine that is less painful and that has no serious side effects.

The nation's only anthrax vaccine, mandatory for most military personnel since 1998, is as safe as any other vaccine and will prevent infection from inhaled spores, concludes an extensive report issued by the Institute of Medicine (IOM) in March 2002. However, the report committee made it clear that the vaccine should be given only to those at high risk for exposure. The anthrax attacks of 2001[1] left some physicians in a quandary when panicked patients demanded the vaccine.

These main conclusions were darkened by the report committee's concern about the vaccine's inadequacies, including an 18-month immunization schedule, painful subcutaneous delivery, and outdated design. Manufactured by Bioport Corp, Lansing, Michigan, the vaccine was developed in the 1950s at Camp Detrik (now Fort Detrick), Maryland, which at the time housed a biological weapons program.

1. In the fall of 2001, envelopes containing anthrax spores were mailed to several media and government addresses, resulting in five deaths.

While fears of attacks from similar weapons prompted the military to adopt the vaccine, the injections were originally meant to ward off anthrax from a much less sinister source—barnyard animals. In fact, the only randomized, placebo-controlled human study, which led to US Food and Drug Administration (FDA) approval in 1970, involved workers at goat-hair mills.

Questions in the military

Decades later, a number of concerned servicemen and servicewomen raised questions about the vaccine they were required to receive. Reports of chronic fatigue-like symptoms, memory loss, suspected links to Gulf War illness (some veterans of that war received the vaccine), and other complaints surfaced after the military's mass vaccination program began. Many refused to be vaccinated against anthrax. The fracas led Congress to direct the IOM to conduct the study, which was expedited after the mail attacks of 2001.

Ideally, a new [anthrax] vaccine would not cause any severe reactions, would require two or three injections instead of six, and would prompt immunity within 30 days.

Despite the high visibility of the vaccine's detractors, the IOM committee found no evidence of serious adverse events. The frequency and type of adverse effects fall within the range considered normal, said committee chair Brian Strom, MD, MPH. Itching and soreness at injection sites, occasional fatigue, and viruslike symptoms all resolved within a few days, according to the committee's review of the Vaccine Adverse Event Reporting System (VAERS), a joint program of the FDA and the Centers for Disease Control and Prevention to monitor all licensed vaccines.

The committee also found that despite limited data, "the available evidence to date does not confirm any long-term health risks. . . ." However, because no vaccine is 100% safe, the committee said, the Department of Defense should create systems to enhance long-term monitoring of health conditions that might be associated with any vaccine given to military personnel.

Reports of serious illnesses such as Guillain-Barre syndrome and atrial fibrillation were very rare and either unrelated to the anthrax vaccine or unclassifiable, concluded the committee. However, they also said that VAERS tends to underestimate the true number of adverse events. The system relies heavily on physician initiative to complete and return forms. Many, even those who care for military patients, simply are not aware of the process or do not bother with it, said committee member Hugh Tilson, MD, DrPH, senior advisor to the dean at the School of Public Health, University of North Carolina, Chapel Hill.

In addition, the report notes that some military vaccinees complained that they had been discouraged from reporting adverse effects: "In at least one Air Force squadron there is a perception that seeking care for symptoms of unknown origin or filing a VAERS report carries the risk of being labeled a malingerer. . . ." The committee found that the US Department of Defense had responded appropriately to the complaints.

All things considered, the concerns ware enough to prompt the committee to make a forceful plea for an improved vaccine. Ideally, a new vaccine would not cause any severe reactions, would require two or three injections instead of six, and would prompt immunity within 30 days that lasts for at least a year. In addition, the report said, any new vaccine needs a long shelf life to ensure ample stockpiles for a worst-case biological attack.

The committee noted that natural mutations or bioengineered alterations in anthrax bacteria would not be apt to produce strains that are vaccine resistant. The vaccine acts directly on a toxin from the bacteria, which must remain unaltered for the bacteria to retain its lethal nature.

12

The Effort to Develop New Vaccines Could Help Prevent War

Peter J. Hotez

Peter J. Hotez is chair of the Department of Microbiology and Tropical Medicine at George Washington University and a senior fellow of the Albert B. Sabin Vaccine Institute, where he is principal investigator of the Human Hookworm Vaccine Initiative.

A multinational effort to eradicate disease through immunization will not only save lives, it could also help reduce global conflicts. Such was the case during the Cold War, when Soviet virologists worked with U.S. researchers to create an improved polio vaccine, and during a mid-1990s civil conflict in Sudan, when a cease-fire was negotiated so that the region could concentrate on reducing a parasitic illness. Today, efforts to develop vaccines that combat tropical diseases could help reduce the possibility of war in South Asia.

Vaccines are arguably one of humankind's greatest creations. Because of vaccines' remarkable ability to halt great plagues and eliminate disease, few other peacetime inventions have had as much influence on human history. Within the last 20 years alone, vaccines have eradicated smallpox, with polio soon to follow. But inoculations that eliminate disease could have an impact well beyond improving global health. Throughout the developing world, vaccines could also be transformed into powerful agents of conflict resolution.

Vaccine diplomacy

Vaccine diplomacy is nearly as old as vaccines themselves. In 1798, British doctor Edward Jenner published his research on the use of the cowpox (vaccinia) virus to vaccinate (from the Latin word for cow) against the human smallpox virus. By 1800, the Jenner smallpox vaccine was used widely in England and shipped across the channel to France. Within a decade, Napoleon decreed that vaccine departments should be established in all of the major cities of the French empire. And in 1811 Jenner was elected as a foreign member of the Institute of France. Strikingly, Jenner's participation in the use and development of the smallpox vaccine in France occurred during a time of almost continuous war between England and France. But, as Jenner himself observed in a letter to the National Institute of France, "The sciences are never at war."

Throughout the developing world, vaccines could . . . be transformed into powerful agents of conflict resolution.

Similarly, in the early 1950s, polio epidemics raged on both sides of the Iron Curtain. The dreadful nature of these epidemics (they struck young children particularly hard) could have been the deciding factor in compelling the Soviets to break their Cold War silence in 1956 when they realized, in the words of medical historian Saul Benison, "they could no longer afford the comfort and sustenance that ideology provided." Soviet virologists subsequently collaborated with U.S. researcher Albert Sabin to develop a "live" polio vaccine that improved upon the one developed by Jonas Salk in 1954. To this day, many Americans are astonished to learn that the Sabin polio vaccine was introduced into the United States only after its safety and efficacy had first been tested in millions of Soviet children.

The legacy of Cold War vaccine diplomacy is now felt in polio-endemic regions of Africa and Central Asia where, since 1996, the United Nations Children's Fund and the World Health Organization have negotiated cease-fires in order to conduct successful polio immunization campaigns. Through the efforts of United Nations agencies, mass vaccinations during so-called days of tranquility have been brokered every year in Afghanistan since 1993. In Sudan, former U.S. President Jimmy Carter helped negotiate a six-month cease-fire in 1995 to reduce the incidence of drancunculiasis, a parasitic disease caused by the guinea worm. (The "guinea worm cease-fire" was, at that time, the longest cease-fire in the history of the Sudanese civil conflict.) National immunization days also temporarily halted hostilities in Sierra Leone.

Today, the part of the world most in need of both vaccines and diplomacy is South Asia. In 1998, the Indian government renewed underground nuclear testing in part because of a perceived threat from China. But India and China share more than a disputed border and expanding nuclear capabilities: These two nations, which together comprise approximately 40 percent of the world's population, also share one of the highest rates of tropical infectious diseases. Illnesses caused by animal parasites living in the human intestine are especially endemic to the region. Diagnostic surveys conducted by the Chinese Ministry of Health between 1988 and 1992 revealed more than 500 million cases of ascariasis (an infection caused by a large intestinal roundworm), 212 million cases of whipworm infection, and 194 million cases of hookworm infection. India is equally plagued by these parasites, which cause devastating problems among both children and adults, especially pregnant women.

The technology exists to make a vaccine to control worms in India and China, but the resources available for this task are pathetically meager. Despite the enormous burdens of disease, both nations still spend much of their scientific budget on the physical and mathematical sciences necessary to develop nuclear arsenals. If these nations diverted even one tenth of their nuclear-weapons budgets to vaccine research, diseases like hookworm might be eradicated in the 21st century. Now is the time to advocate a new peace-time mission for the Chinese and Indian scientific communities—to shift their intellects and their resources to eradicating the infections that currently trap their rural citizens in a perpetual cycle of poverty. As Sonia Gandhi, the leader of the Congress Party (and daughter-in-law of former Prime Minister Indira Gandhi), remarked, "science should be used for removing poverty and backwardness in the country."

A multilateral vaccine development program that focuses on tropical infectious diseases highly endemic to South and East Asia might foster a spirit of regional cooperation. Such a program would draw scientists and government health officials from countries engaged in nuclear saber rattling together for a common cause. Moreover, this effort could serve as a model to cope with the next health crisis that will soon ravage the region. Although much of the media coverage of HIV/AIDS has focused on Africa, a newer and possibly more frightening HIV/AIDS epidemic has started to roll through densely populated areas of the Indian subcontinent and China. Through government agencies and private foundations, developed countries can commit critical resources to accelerate the development of new vaccines. Along the way, we might acquire an immunity to war.

Organizations to Contact

The editors have compiled the following list of organizations concerned with the issues debated in this book. The descriptions are derived form materials provided by the organizations. All have publications or information available for interested readers. The list was compiled on the date of publication of the present volume; the information provided here may change. Be aware that many organizations take several weeks or longer to respond to inquiries, so allow as much time as possible.

American Council on Science and Health (ACSH)
1995 Broadway, 2nd Fl., New York, NY 10023-5860
(212) 362-7044 • fax: (212) 362-4919
website: www.acsh.org

ACSH is a consumer education consortium concerned with, among other topics, issues related to health and disease. ACSH publishes *Priorities* magazine and position papers such as *Facts Versus Fears: A Review of the Greatest Unfounded Health Scares of Recent Times*.

Centers for Disease Control and Prevention (CDC)
1600 Clifton Rd., Atlanta, GA 30333
(404) 639-3311 • Immunization Hotline (800) 232-2522
website: www.cdc.gov

The CDC is the government agency charged with protecting the public health of the nation by preventing and controlling diseases and by responding to public health emergencies. Programs of the CDC include the National Center for Infectious Diseases, which publishes *Addressing Emerging Infectious Disease Threats: A Prevention Strategy for the United States* and the journal *Emerging Infectious Diseases*. The CDC website includes an index of links to fact sheets, frequently asked questions, press releases, and articles on diseases, vaccines, and immunization.

Federation of American Scientists
Program for Monitoring Emerging Diseases (ProMED)
307 Massachusetts Ave. NE, Washington, DC 20002
(202) 675-1011 • fax: (202) 675-1010
e-mail: dpreslan@fas.org • website: www.fas.org

The Federation of American Scientists is a privately funded, nonprofit organization engaged in analysis and advocacy on science, technology, and public policy for global security. ProMED seeks to link scientists, public health officials, journalists, and laypersons in a global communications network for reporting disease outbreaks. The federation requests that students and other researchers first investigate the resources available on its website, such as the papers *Controlling Infectious Diseases* and *Global Monitoring of Emerging Diseases: Design for a Demonstration Program*, before requesting further information.

Food and Drug Administration (FDA)
5600 Fishers Ln., Rockville, MD 20857
(888) 463-6332
website: www.fda.org

Part of the U.S. Department of Health and Human Services, the FDA's mission is to promote and protect the public health by helping safe and effective foods, drugs, and medicines reach the market in a timely manner, and to monitor such products for continued safety after they are in use. The administration's work is a blending of law and science aimed at protecting consumers. The FDA publishes the magazine *FDA Consumer* as well as fact sheets and updates on vaccine safety, effectiveness, and availability.

Global Vaccine Awareness League (GVAL)
25422 Trabuco Rd., Suite 105-230, Lake Forest, CA 92630-2797
e-mail: Michelle@gval.com • website: www.gval.com

The league is a nonprofit organization committed to educating parents and concerned citizens about the potential risks and serious side effects of vaccines. It publishes a newsletter, fact sheets about vaccines, books, videotapes, and pamphlets such as *Exemption Information for U.S. States* and *Disease—The Power That Heals the Body.*

National Coalition for Adult Immunization
4733 Bethesda Ave., Suite 750, Bethesda, MD 20814-5288
(301) 656-0003 • fax: (301) 907-0878
e-mail: ncai@nfid.org • website: www.nfid.org

The NCAI is a nonprofit organization composed of more than ninety-five professional medical and health care associations, advocacy groups, voluntary organizations, vaccine manufacturers, and government health agencies. The common goal of all members is to improve the immunization status of adults and adolescents to levels specified by the U.S. Public Health Service. Annually, the NCAI publishes the *Resource Guide for Adult and Adolescent Immunization* and spearheads the National Adult Immunization Awareness Week campaign in October. The organization also publishes a newsletter and papers such as *A Call to Action: Improving Influenza and Pneumococcal Immunization Rates Among High-Risk Adults* and *Standards for Adult Immunization Practice.*

National Foundation for Infectious Diseases (NFID)
4733 Bethesda Ave., Suite 750, Bethesda, MD 20814
(301) 656-0003 • fax: (301) 907-0878
e-mail: info@nfid.org • website: www.nfid.org

The foundation is a nonprofit philanthropic organization that supports disease research through grants and fellowships and educates the public about research, treatment, and prevention of infectious diseases. It publishes a newsletter, *Double Helix*, and its website contains a "Virtual Library of Diseases."

National Institute of Allergy and Infectious Diseases (NIAID)
Vaccine Research Center, Building 40, Room 4502, 31 Center Dr. MSC 2520, Bethesda, MD 20892-2520
(301) 496-1852 • fax: (301) 496-5717
e-mail: gnable@nih.gov • website: www.niaid.nih.gov

The institute, one of the programs of the National Institutes of Health, supports scientists conducting research on infectious, immunologic, and allergic diseases that afflict people worldwide. Vaccines and emerging diseases consti-tute two of the NIAID's main areas of research, and many materials are avail-able from the NIAID on these topics, including *Understanding Vaccines* and *Emerging Infectious Diseases Research: Meeting the Challenge*. The website in-cludes a searchable database with links to articles on diseases, vaccine re-search, and bioterrorism.

National Vaccine Information Center (NVIC)
421-E Church St., Vienna, VA 22180
(800) 909-7468 • (703) 938-0342 • fax: (703) 938-5768
website: www.909shot.com

Founded in 1982, the NVIC is the oldest and largest parent-led organization dedicated to the prevention of vaccine injuries and deaths through public ed-ucation. The center provides assistance to parents whose children have suf-fered vaccine reactions and promotes research to evaluate vaccine safety and effectiveness as well as to identify factors which place individuals at high risk for suffering vaccine reactions. The NVIC supports the right of citizens to ex-ercise informed consent and make educated, independent vaccination deci-sions for themselves and their children. The center distributes information on vaccine safety and on reporting adverse effects after vaccination, and it pub-lishes the book *The Consumer's Guide to Childhood Vaccines*.

Bibliography

Books

Harold E. Buttram	*The Immune Trio: Dangers of Immunization, How to Legally Avoid Immunization, and Vaccinations and Immune Malfunction.* Quakertown, PA: Humanitarian Publishing Company, 1996.
Stephanie Cave and Deborah Mitchell	*What Your Doctor May Not Tell You About Children's Vaccinations.* New York: Warner Books, 2001.
Leonard A. Cole	*The Eleventh Plague: The Politics of Biological and Chemical Warfare.* New York: W.H. Freeman, 1997.
Henry Gabowski and John Vernon	*The Search for New Vaccines: The Effects of the Vaccines for Children Program.* Washington, DC: AEI Press, 1997.
George C. Kohn	*Encyclopedia of Plague and Pestilence: From Ancient Times to the Present,* Revised Edition. New York: Facts On File, 2002.
Gary Null and James Feast	*Germs, Biological Warfare, Vaccinations: What You Need to Know.* New York: Seven Stories Press, 2002.
Nicholas Regush	*The Virus Within: A Coming Epidemic.* New York: Plume, 2001.
Hazel Richardson	*Killer Diseases.* New York: Dorling Kindersley, 2002.
Aviva Jill Romm	*Vaccinations: A Thoughtful Parent's Guide—How to Make Safe, Sensible Decisions About the Risks, Benefits, and Alternatives.* Rochester, VT: Healing Arts Press, 2001.
Diane Rozario	*The Immunization Resource Guide: Where to Find Answers to All Your Questions About Childhood Vaccinations.* Burlington, IA: Patter Publications, 2001.

Periodicals

Arthur Allen	"Injection Rejection: The Dangerous Backlash Against Vaccination," *New Republic,* March 23, 1998.
Haroon Ashraf	"U.S. Expert Group Rejects Link Between MMR and Autism," *The Lancet,* April 28, 2001.
Douglas S. Barasch	"How Safe Are Kids' Vaccines?" *Good Housekeeping,* September 2000.
Robert Breiman	"Vaccines as Tools for Advancing More than Public Health: Perspectives of a Former Director of the National Vaccine Program Office," *Clinical Infectious Diseases,* January 15, 2001.

David Brown   "Precious Ounces of Prevention," *Washington Post National Weekly Edition,* April 29–May 5, 2002.

Business Week   "Why Vaccines Are Our Best Shot: They're the Most Effective Way to Deal with Diseases Like Anthrax and Smallpox . . ." October 18, 2001.

Victoria Stagg Elliott "Polio Nearly Gone; Should Vaccine End Too?" *American Medical News,* January 14, 2002.

Karen Engberg   "Vaccinations Keep Children Out of Harms' Way," *Philadelphia Inquirer,* February 25, 1997.

Carolyn Gard   "How Vaccines Work: A Little Pain in the Arm Now Eliminates a Lot of Pain Later," *Current Health,* November 2001.

Steve Goldstein   "Weapon Counterterrorism Officials Fear Most Is Smallpox," *Philadelphia Inquirer,* March 31, 2000.

Melissa Meyers   "A Shot in the Arm," *Men's Health,* January/February
Gotthardt   1996.

Kathleen M. Heins   "Childhood Vaccines," *Better Homes and Gardens,* October 2000.

Aimee Howd   "When Vaccines Do Harm to Kids," *Insight on the News,* February 28, 2000.

Lynn McTaggart   "Doctor's Handwriting," *The Ecologist,* March 2001.

Maryann Napoli   "The Possible Link Between MMR Vaccine and Autism: An Interview with Barbara Loe Fisher," *Healthfacts,* December 2000.

Susan Okie   "The Smallpox Tradeoff," *Washington Post National Weekly Edition,* May 13–19, 2002.

Kelly Patricia O'Meara "Inoculations May Be Rx for Disaster," *Insight on the News,* October 4, 1999.

Wendy Orent   "Cattle Call: Where to Find an Anthrax Vaccine," *New Republic,* November 12, 2001.

Stanley A. Plotkin,   "The Eradication of Rubella," *JAMA,* February 10, 1999.
Michael Katz, and
Jose F. Cordero

David A. Salmon et al. "Health Consequences of Religious and Philosophical Exemptions from Immunization Laws," *JAMA,* July 7, 1999.

Edmund Sanders   "U.S. Weighs Risk of Smallpox, and Risk of Smallpox Vaccine," *Los Angeles Times,* June 16, 2002.

Spectator   "MMR Saves Lives," February 9, 2002.

Miriam E. Tucker   "Multiple Vaccines Not Tied to Immune Dysfunction," *Pediatric News,* February 2002.

Vaccine Weekly   "Report Supports Infant Vaccinations," April 17, 2002.

Andrew Weil and   "The Vaccination Debate: Modern Miracle or Time
Richard Moskowitz   Bomb?" *Natural Health,* November/December 1997.

Elizabeth M. Whelan   "Don't Panic. We Can Fight Smallpox," *Wall Street Journal,* October 25, 2001.

John A.T. Young and   "Attacking Anthrax," *Scientific American,* March 2002.
R. John Collier

Index